SURVIVING PTSD & MORAL INJURY

HOW AN AFGHANISTAN VETERAN BREAKS THE
SILENCE ON MENTAL ILLNESS

ERIK KRIKKE

Title: *Surviving PTSD & moral injury. How an Afghanistan veteran breaks the silence on mental illness*

Author: Erik Krikke

ISBN 13: 9789492371546 (ebook)

ISBN 13: 9789492371539 (paperback)

Publisher: Amsterdam Publishers

Cover photos: Willemijn de Vries

Translation: Ilona Rysavy Patchesa

Original Dutch title: *Operatie Geslaagd. Afghanistan: van oorlogschirurgie naar PTSS*, Boekscout, April 2016 (ISBN paperback 9789402229363, ISBN hardcover 9789402232202)

I dedicate this book to all of those who didn't return from their mission, and to them who did return, but for whom the burden got too heavy to bear.

Lest we forget.

CONTENTS

RECOMMENDATION

"Round the clock assisting in war surgery got to him. He went from aid worker to victim when he was confronted by his PTSD some years later. This realistic book shows his battle and how he got back up after he hit rock bottom. I am proud of him." – General Tom Middendorp, Netherlands Chief of Defence (ret.)

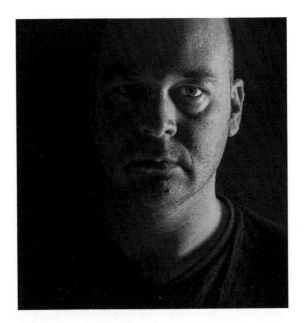

Erik Krikke (2017)

RELIVING

The screams of the patient are blood-curdling. The police car he was travelling in hit a landmine. The attack happened just a few miles away from our camp. I suddenly realise that the blast we heard earlier this morning almost certainly was the explosion of this mine.

The hospital slowly fills with the now familiar scent that every victim of an explosion seems to be carrying: a sickening mixture of diesel, gunpowder, blood and burnt flesh.

"My legs," the young policeman mutters over and over again, "don't take them off. Please, don't take them off. Without my legs I won't be able to live."

His right leg is severely damaged. It is positioned in an unnatural angle below the knee. His trousers have been torn to pieces and the left leg doesn't look much better. The rest of his body is covered in a grey layer of sand, dust and dried blood. It is obvious that he won't be going out on patrol ever again.

At the same time another patient is carried to the hospital. With every step the stretcher crew takes, his head bobs powerlessly from side to side. The stretcher is placed in front of the hospital's door. As soon as it touches the floor, his head drops back and his arms spread out. His eyes are half-open and it is as though he is staring up to the sky, wondering what has happened to him. There is no light in his eyes anymore; he is beyond help.

~

Our bedroom is pitch-black. I wake up with a shock. Gasping for air I sit upright in bed and look around wildly. It seems to take ages before I realise that I am safely tucked up in bed. I am not in Afghanistan anymore, I am home. As I repeat these words over and over in my head, like a mantra, they don't seem ring true.

I glance over to my wife next to me who is sound asleep. Her regular breathing tells me she hasn't noticed a thing. Thank goodness. I am so ashamed. All my senses are heightened. I am soaking wet from the sweat, but I feel cold as ice at the same time. As tears fall down my cheeks, I try to suppress a feeling of nausea, triggered by a scent that is rooted deep within my brain. It is the scent of death.

Quietly I get out of bed and make my way to the bathroom. I switch on the light, grab the sink with both hands and look up slowly. As I look in the mirror, my eyes meet the eyes of a total stranger and I can't help to feel sorry for him. The pain I see in his hollow eyes gets to me. Then I recognise him.

I stumble to a corner in the bathroom and curl up. With my arms wrapped tightly around my knees I sit there for ages. My mind is racing. I don't want this anymore. Why the hell did I let it get to this?

A warm hand on my forearm and a soft voice suddenly startle me. "Daddy, why are you crying?"

INTRODUCTION

Ten years ago, I flew out to Afghanistan to work as a military operating room nurse at Kandahar Airfield. During my deployment I helped to save the lives and limbs of many severely wounded victims and it turned out to be a period that would radically change my life.

Even though my wounds aren't visible, I have had to fight hard to get to where I am now, to survive. To not become one of the many for whom the battle became too much.

In front of you is my story about the experiences that have led to my PTSD and my fight against it. The hardest battle I have ever had to fight in my life: the one against my memories, but above all with myself.

Writing about it has not been easy at all. I am sharing my story with you to raise awareness of working through trauma and PTSD. One doesn't have PTSD on their own. Partners, family and friends fight just as hard alongside of the one suffering from it.

~

I made it with the help of my family, friends and professionals. Because of them I can now live my life to the full again. Nowadays, I can and want to talk about it to help others. This would not have been possible, and I could not have come this far without their support and love.

I tell my story in this book, but I also do that on stage. With my band I tour theatres to tell about it through music. Break the silence? Yes, absolutely!

The development of my PTSD can be compared to a physical wound that I refused treatment for. Instead of having immediate surgery I covered it up. It became inflamed and an abscess developed under the skin, which burst years later. I looked for help and found it. The wound got opened up again and a lengthy procedure was needed to remove all the crap, and also to prevent it from ever happening again. The wound was left open to help it heal from the inside out and from deep within. All that is left now is a scar that is still red, inflamed and ugly, but which will fade away in time. It is still sore at times, but it won't rip open again.

I have made huge steps. Much too late, but I am on the right track and I am now able to do something positive with it all.

I got rid of most of the ghosts from the past. I used to suffer from reliving memories, flashbacks, and nightmares, and I even used to worry about the sense and nonsense of carrying on with living, but it is as if a switch has been flipped.

I did away with the pathological coping mechanisms I used for years. I always thought I could do it all on my own, but could not have been more wrong. More than once I have had a rude awakening. Like so many people, I grew up with the idea that I am man enough to handle everything on my own. I always used to be there for everyone, but I never held out my hand for it to be taken by someone who could help me. I have learned from that.

One fateful summer in Afghanistan has changed my life forever. What I saw, heard, smelt, tasted and felt there, has shaken me to the core. I thought I would be able to keep going by avoiding and escaping, but that was a mistake. Even though I managed to keep going for a while, I eventually hit a wall and I am sure I am not the only one.

PTSD gets under people's skin, waiting for the most vulnerable moment to suddenly strike. There have been days during which I couldn't see it getting any better and when I wanted to stop my treatment to bury my head in the sand again. I am pleased that I have been strong enough to keep fighting, and that I still am.

What I most resent myself for, is that I refused to look for help for such a long time. Multiple roads, both within the armed forces and elsewhere, lead to help. I was so stupid to keep holding on to my own mantra of being able to manage it all on my own.

The water was up to my neck. I had to nearly drown before I dared to ask for a lifeline. I had to feel completely numb, both at home and at work, before I dared to look in the mirror and admit I wasn't well. For years I tried to build a wall around myself, but it wasn't strong enough, and it finally collapsed.

PTSD will always be there. It lays dormant in my system and rears its head when it is most inconvenient. Bit by bit though, it seems to become manageable.

Where I used to live day by day, and couldn't predict in the morning whether it was going to be a good or a bad day, I now live in a more structured way. I no longer go from the highest highs to the lowest lows and back again. Days are much better and some are simply good.

I still grieve regularly, and I am not sure if that will ever go away. It is okay for that to happen. All of my experiences have made me the person I am today. I have grown as a human being. I just chose the difficult way to get there.

What has helped me immensely through all of this misery is structure. That was the first piece of advice I was given: make sure your life is structured and start small, with a solid daily routine. Housework, walking, fitness and judo were my daily routine. On top of that I started writing down my experiences and feelings in detail. The latter made me experience the deployment again in all its gruesome detail.

War surgery is a discipline in its own right.

I was ashamed that we weren't always able to offer the care we wanted to. I was also ashamed about amputating people's limbs who would probably be condemned to a life of beggary. Patients who begged us not to amputate their legs and told us they would rather die. I didn't feel proud at all of what I did during my deployment.

As I slowly opened up to people around me about working in an operating room during the war, they would tell me how much they respected me for that. I have found out how important it is to talk to people close to you.

Recognition and pride. They are both vague concepts I didn't really understand veterans could actually experience, as I felt a total lack of both of them. Only after lots of talking, and sharing everything with the people around me, I sometimes experience what they actually mean.

I get a lot of reactions to my story and almost every one speaks of respect. All of this helps me to retrieve my lost pride.

～

Asking for help is not a sign of weakness. On the contrary, it is a sign of strength. It was the hardest decision to make, years after my deployment. I knew that I let tension build up over six years, and had to admit I couldn't handle it on my own anymore.

The moment that I picked up the phone and rang the Veterans Institute was one of the most difficult moments of my life, because I realised I had a problem and I had to admit it. During that tough and emotional phone call the armed forces told me they would be my safety net and I am glad to say that they have kept their word.

I am still under treatment. The PTSD and moral injury will be a part of my life forever. I have changed permanently, but that is okay, and I simply let the bad days happen. I don't fight them anymore.

The fear of my memories is slowly but surely fading away. There will be one last confrontation in the future, as I will return to where it all began. Together with my psychologist I will go back to Kandahar for some sort of Proper Exit and to retrieve the piece of me that I left there.

~

I do as many fun things as possible, since they give me positive energy to keep going. I do that for and with myself, my family and my friends and I will show everyone that I continue to cope with PTSD, even though one day might be better than the next.

The switch is flipped; I no longer flee, I fight. I have been in our house for years, but I have never actually come home. I have been ready to give it all up, but thanks to the help and support of my therapists within the armed forces, and my family, friends and fellow veterans I am on my way back. I continue to climb this mountain.

Although the top is still shrouded in mist, I know it is there in the distance. I will undoubtedly stumble and slide down a bit during the ascent, but I am not giving up until I have reached the top.

Only then my mission will be accomplished.

CHANGING OUR HOLIDAY PLANS

In February 2007 I am asked to go and see the head of the surgery department of the hospital where I work.

I know what is coming. Cursing loudly I down the last sip of my cold, weak hospital coffee and walk reluctantly to his office. It has been talked about for quite some time now. A surgical team from our hospital is going to be deployed in Afghanistan.

Because a couple of my colleagues have recently retired and some others have been transferred, my name has quickly moved up to second place on the operating room nurses' list. As two of us will be deployed, I now have to start preparing myself for a trip to Afghanistan.

Many of my colleagues see a deployment as one big adventure and as the jewel in the crown of their work in the armed forces. I see it like that too, but since the birth of my two children I have turned into a real family man. I prefer to be at home every night. I am a daddy who is almost certainly serving his final contract. I have been thinking of leaving at the end of my current contract for a while now.

My conversation with the head of surgery consists of a brief, businesslike summary of what is to come and is, at the same time, the official appointment for the mission. It feels like I have just been sentenced. I am going to spend the entire summer in the Afghan desert.

I am off to the Role 3 MMU (*Multinational Medical Unit*), the NATO hospital at the huge military base at Kandahar Airfield (KAF) in the south of Afghanistan. I need to tell my wife that we will have to change our holiday plans.

The Role 3 hospital has the resources to thoroughly diagnose and treat patients and also has the capacity to perform surgeries. It is under command of the Canadian Armed Forces. Apart from Canadians, the hospital is run by military personnel from several coalition countries. Our contribution consists of, amongst other things, supplying a surgical team. The team that I am going to be part of includes an orthopaedic surgeon, an anaesthetist, a nurse anaesthetist and two operating room nurses, or OR nurses.

I will be working as one of the OR nurses at the hospital's surgery department. All victims the war throws up in the southern part of Afghanistan will be sent here. Our task will be to perform surgical intervention in order to save lives.

After my appointment I read up a bit on the history of the country. I didn't know much more about Afghanistan than what was shown on the news. It is common knowledge that it is an unsettled country and that there are many incidents with IEDs (*Improvised Explosive Devices*), which make a lot of casualties amongst both coalition troops and the Afghan forces.

I have seen images of the damage such a bomb can cause to a human body. There are regular suicide attacks, which also claim lots of civilian victims. I try to imagine what it will be like.

~

At home I tell my wife Harriette in a few words that I have been appointed earlier that day. The news doesn't come as a complete surprise, as I had told her before that my name was climbing up the list. A short discussion follows. She explains that she is really not happy and struggles with the fact that I will be gone for such a long time as the kids are still so young.

Our sons Mika and Lars are only four and nearly three years old. I tell her I feel the same, but that we both know that it is part of my job. We sit silently opposite each other at the kitchen table, both deep in thought. I look at our playing children and then I look up. My eyes find hers.

"We'll have to get rid of the dog," I say out of the blue. To break the awkward silence, I switch to practical mode.

My wife looks at me with a puzzled look on her face.

Then I see her slowly coming back down to earth.

"Yes, I think you might be right," she says.

Our dog is a Rottweiler / Labrador cross and since the births of our sons he has changed from a tail-wagging friend to a moody, growling guard dog. I simply don't dare to leave my family alone with him. I would never be able to forgive myself if the animal grabs one of the children whilst I am away. A few days later we make a decision. We take the dog away.

To prepare for deployment, I attend a course focussing on the mission. Our surgical team takes part in it and the team that will be taking over from us after our deployment is also present.

The programme includes informative talks about Afghanistan. Especially practical matters are discussed. We are instructed on the climate and the importance of acclimatising. We also receive information about the flora and fauna in Afghanistan, and about diseases known to exist in the country, such as malaria, tuberculosis and *cutaneous leishmaniasis* (a skin infection caused by a parasite that is transmitted by tiny mosquitoes, also known as sand flies).

Cultural background and media training also form part of the programme, and we discuss possible decompression days during our return journey. After the operational deployment there will be a stopover in Crete to undergo a transition period of several days. After working under high levels of stress, it is useful to relax for a couple of days before returning home. This is to prevent that deployed individuals stay in survival mode. It is immediately stated though that it is not sure we will actually be considered for these days.

There are lectures and presentations by medical personnel who have already been deployed to Kandahar. We get to see pictures of the hospital, and also of casualties with blown-off limbs. From a strictly professional point of view this summer could well turn out to be a very interesting time. Looking at the pictures I assume that we will see these sorts of injuries occasionally. My colleague Linda though seems somewhat distressed, as she expects the exact opposite and envisages that we will come across these horrific injuries all the time. Even before the mission our expectations are poles apart.

The main part of the presentations during our instruction week focusses on non-essential issues. Kandahar Airfield is a huge base and it has lots of facilities, ranging from. mobile fast-food chains like Burger King, Subway and Pizza Hut to coffee chains like Green Beans and Tim Hortons. There are also a few duty-free shops and apparently there is even a massage salon.

Because of these presentations, an idyllic picture of an all-inclusive sun holiday forms in my head. But despite all the aforementioned comforts it is still a tour to a Taliban stronghold. This summer we will be travelling to the southern Afghan desert. The weather will be hot;

I quickly dismiss the thought that the situation is heating up over there too.

We will be working in a war hospital with the people and means available over there; it is going to be a challenge. I hold on to the fact that I will undoubtedly come home with a nice tan and a wealth of experience.

HOMECARE

My imminent deployment is a major event, not just for me but also for my wife and children.

During the buildup we have some intense discussions at home. They are mostly about people's reactions to the news of my appointment. My family for example are very levelheaded. "He'll be back in no time. Those few months are nothing at all, are they now?"

Every time someone utters these words, I notice something in Harriette's eyes. It is as if she wants to say something, but then decides against it. I don't ask her what she is thinking.

The day I am due to leave is approaching fast. I sort out lots of practical things, we do some bulk grocery shopping and both of us take an afternoon off to have our family's pictures taken. I solemnly swear that I will put them up above my bed in Kandahar as soon as I get there.

The final bit of preparation is something I have been putting off till the last minute. There is a pile of paperwork to fill in, including the *Next of Kin Handbook*, which is exactly what it sounds like. In case I come home in a box, this manual explains everything that needs to be arranged according to my last wishes.

Completing this paperwork is confrontational, as I have to deliberately think about a subject no one actually wants to think about. After all, dying during deployment only 'happens to others.'

The same goes for PTSD, *Post-Traumatic Stress Disorder*, or a burn-out. I won't ever let that happen to myself. I am a big, down-to-earth, well-balanced guy and I have managed just fine all my life. That is exactly how it will stay. On the last day before leaving, I lock myself in my office and fill in the manual. It takes me hours. I choose music for my funeral, decide who should and shouldn't receive an announcement of my passing and commit more personal wishes to paper too. When I am finished I feel tired and dejected. As I have been so focussed on death whilst filling in this paperwork, I now realise that my 'holiday in the sun' will be a risky one. I tell my wife that I will leave it all in a sealed envelope in my office and I promise her that we will get rid of it as soon as I return.

The fact that daddy is leaving for such a long time is a big thing in our children's lives and that is why I spend as much time as I can with them in the period before my deployment.

I stick a large calendar on the cupboard, which starts on the day of my departure and finishes on the expected day of return. Next to it is a huge jar filled with as many sweets for both boys as there are days on the calendar. I tell them that they are allowed to have one sweet a day. This means they will see the jar empty day by day. They will cross off the days on the calendar in a way they understand and is yummy at the same time.

"When you have eaten all the sweets, Daddy will be home again," I tell them.

My wife and I have intentionally put a lot more sweets in the jar than we needed to. We have also added more days to the calendar than my deployment is supposed to take, just in case there is an unexpected delay.

"Mika and Lars, remember, one per person per day. There is no point in stuffing yourselves as soon as I have stepped onto the aircraft. That won't make me come home any sooner. All it will do is give you tummy ache."

It takes one to know one.

~

"Daddy is leaving this afternoon. I'll miss you, boys. Will you miss me too?" I look from one to the other and their smiles warm my heart. Then both of them wrap themselves around me at the same time. I hold them tight and try to fight my tears as best as I can.

My wife and I take our youngest son, Lars, to pre-school, where I give him one last kiss and cuddle. Then he runs to the group of children and starts to play without a care in the world. His pre-school teacher joins us for a moment and wishes me, but also my wife, good luck. As soon as she says those words, my wife starts to cry quietly. I quickly say goodbye and take her outside.

After we have dropped off Lars, we take Mika to school. As a final goodbye I give him a kiss and a big hug. He looks back one more time and gives me a big smile before he strolls into school.

"I love you," I say as I wave him off. I stay at the playground for just that bit longer. A lot of the other parents look at us and it is as if no one actually dares to say anything. I don't mind, I don't feel like talking anyway. Dressed in my desert gear I take my wife by the hand and we leave the playground in a hurry.

We have decided she won't come to the airport to wave me off. Harriette has made it clear that she won't be able to handle that and we both don't want to have a tearful farewell. That is why my parents will take me.

After an intense goodbye at home I get in the car. I quickly drive to a really good friend of mine. I am always welcome at his house for a cup of coffee, a silly joke and a firm handshake.

"Keep your head down," he advises.

I promise to do exactly that, say my goodbyes and drive to my parents so we can go to the airport together. The journey is about to begin.

The departure lounge at the airbase is filled with people saying goodbye to their loved ones, family and friends. There is laughter and tears, people hug like it is the last time. I meet up with my team members and say goodbye to my parents. I feel that my mum has suddenly aged beyond her years. I kiss her and tell her everything will be fine. I can see her fighting her tears as I do that.

"Don't worry, mum, you know me."

"Yes, I do, Erik, that's why." Although she is smiling, I can see the sorrow in her eyes.

After a little while we get a call telling us that it is time to check in and to get ourselves ready for departure. I quickly ring Harriette one last time to tell her how much I love her. Then I go outside to smoke a final cigarette and walk through the gate.

THE START OF A JOURNEY

We left three days ago, early in the evening. In a huge transport plane we were supposed to fly to our first stop Kabul, the capital of Afghanistan. The plan was that we would be flown from there to Kandahar, our final destination. Almost immediately the journey didn't go as planned. The Iranian authorities hadn't granted us permission to enter their airspace, so we had to make a stopover in Turkey. A new flight plan had to be submitted the next day so we could continue on to Kabul International Airport.

We landed at Kabul early in the morning and stayed at a heavily guarded part of the airport, where we had to wait to hear when we would get flown to our final destination Kandahar.

We received our weapons. I put the clips with cartridges away and I put my gun, a Glock 17, in the holster on my right leg. From then on, I would feel its weight with every step I would take. We were also supplied with our helmets and flak jackets, which we would have to wear during the last part of our trip. Now that I was armed, I realised we had entered a war zone.

The rest of the day we spent at the airport where we took some time to visit the hospital. Only two patients had been admitted and personnel at the hospital told us it had been really quiet in and around Kabul for the past few weeks.

For most of the day we were hanging out at the Holland House, a nicely furnished building with lots of orange elements. We didn't have to wait long to find out more about the next part of our journey. We would leave for Kandahar that night.

During the last part of the trip we would be transported in a tactical transport plane of the Royal Air Force. I put on my helmet and flak jacket and boarded the C-130 Hercules, which was waiting for us with rotating propellers.

~

All the lights in the transport plane suddenly turn off, apart from a tiny green one. The last phase of the long trip to Kandahar has finally started. Everyone is huddled together and strapped in their safety belts on hard, narrow benches along the side walls of the plane. The rest of the cargo bay is filled with roll pallets packed with goods. Everyone is wearing a flak jacket and a helmet and is holding a weapon firmly between the knees. We are propped up against each other like fish in a barrel. Because of the plane's buffeting and sharp turns, our helmets keep bumping against each other. It looks funny. One half of the passengers are alert and look around tensely, whilst the other half is asleep, their heads hanging low.

This C-130 Hercules is relatively slow. The plane makes tight turns to make it as difficult as possible for potential attackers.

Suddenly, the nose of the plane tilts downwards sharply and the descent begins. The landing is a so-called tactical landing. This means that the plane approaches from great height and only at the last moment the nose comes down to start a steep descent. The manoeuvre makes me feel as if all my intestines abruptly swap places.

It is clear I am not the only one who feels like this, as a few empty the contents of their stomachs into a hastily grabbed paper bag.

With a jolt the plane's wheels touch down on the concrete of Kandahar Airfield.

Kandahar is Afghanistan's second largest city after the capital of Kabul. Kandahar, which is in the southeast, is the capital of the county with which it shares its name and has approximately 391,000 inhabitants. We have travelled over 3,500 miles to get here.

After landing at Kandahar Airfield the cargo door opens and the roll pallets with goods are offloaded first. Slowly everybody frees themselves from their safety belts and gets up. All helmets are levelled, weapons picked up and flak jackets straightened.

When I step off the plane, the desert heat envelops me, although it is nearly midnight. I take my first steps on the concrete runway of Kandahar Airfield and take a quick look around.

"Welcome to the camp that gets shot at most in the whole of Afghanistan!" a surly looking English sergeant major shouts at us when we, one by one, waggle off the plane. His voice needs to rise above the noise of the propellers which are still rotating, but he doesn't seem to have any trouble with that.

His words still echo in my head when I lie in my sleeping bag in a big tent some hours later. I wonder whether I have perhaps been dropped off at the wrong location, because with just that one sentence the Englishman turned the image I had in my mind of Kandahar Airfield on its head.

IRON MAN

The coming weeks I will be part of the surgical team and we will be working closely together with Canadian and American personnel. We will be on standby at the hospital to perform life- and limb saving surgery on injured people who are brought in and need our immediate help.

Whilst days at the surgical department at home are fully organised through a pre-planned surgery programme, the period that is about to start will be totally different. We will perform surgeries as they are presented to us. The patients will literally fall from the sky as most of them will be flown in by helicopter. They will often be on our operating table more than once, because many will need multiple surgeries.

Within any hospital, the OR (operating room) is the one place that always speaks to people's imagination. During a procedure the surgical team is dressed in sterile gowns and everyone wears sterile gloves. Hair is covered up with a surgical cap and faces are mostly hidden by a mask and safety glasses. One glance through the window of an OR door will give the onlooker the feeling that a sacred ritual is being performed. This image would be seriously disrupted if they would set foot in the operating theatre where they would be greeted by deafening heavy metal music and hear doctors and nurses singing along.

The work of an OR nurse is not just a profession, it is also a calling. It is a multifaceted occupation that does not just exist of handing over surgical instruments. This particular image has wrongly generated the nickname *iron man*. An OR nurse helps the surgeon before, during and after the operation. He is the one responsible for making sure the OR is ready to be used for surgery, including all equipment, instruments and other supplies. Supporting patients and reporting form important parts of a surgical assistant's duties. During any surgery the job consists of three main tasks: passing surgical instruments, circulating and assisting.

Passing surgical instruments is also jokingly described as passing cutlery. Whilst being in charge of it, the OR nurse makes sure the surgeon is passed instruments, suture kits and other sterile tools in the correct order at the right time. The person in charge of the instruments stands at the operating table together with the surgeon and is also dressed in sterile clothing.

The OR nurse acts as the surgeon's right-hand man, helps during the procedure and makes sure that the surgeon can, without being interrupted, complete all steps of surgery. The assistant therefore needs to know the procedure and understand which complications could occur.

Circulating is performed by a second OR nurse dressed in non-sterile clothing present at the operating theatre. He manages the extra materials, making sure these are handed over to the sterile team when needed, operates the equipment in the OR and ensures that sterility is maintained at all times. The circulator also takes care of the paperwork relating the surgery.

This is why there are usually two or three OR nurses present in the

OR during surgery. Together with the surgeon, the anaesthetist and the nurse anaesthetist they form a surgical team.

Every OR nurse needs to know the sequence of all steps of every operation, and needs to be familiar with what equipment and other supplies are required and how to use these. Assisting during surgery happens in all specialities. That is why an extensive knowledge of anatomy (the way the body is structured), and physiology (the way the body functions) is important. Any OR nurse has a vast knowledge of every stage of surgery, and of the surgical techniques. All these facets make for varied work. No two days are ever the same.

The work of an OR nurse in Kandahar would require even more flexibility, because not all specialisms are represented at the hospital. There are only a handful of surgeons and they will have to perform surgeries on any patient that comes in. On top of all of this we would have to deal with limited resources and we would need to be as creative as possible to achieve the best outcome under primitive circumstances.

WORKING IN A CABIN

Hovel and plywood. Those words spring to mind when I see the hospital for the first time. "Typical, just my luck. I deploy to Afghanistan and end up in a cabin." The words come out of my mouth before I even realise.

The airport and immense military base Kandahar Airfield is only a couple of miles away from the former Taliban capital Kandahar. The hospital is a collection of windowless boxes made of plywood. It is a mishmash of walls and partitions, and some connected tents and containers. The core of it looks like a hastily built and half-finished shed. The extra containers and tents seem to be added at a later date.

The Role 3 hospital is right next to the taxiway which has the runway behind it. Across from the runway are the plains which extend to the foot of a steep, barren and ragged mountain ridge.

The hospital is enclosed by three-metre-high *blast-walls,* walls made of reinforced concrete stopping shrapnel coming in during a missile attack. These were often fired from the steep mountain ridge mentioned before. The roof is covered with unarmoured plywood. When it rains heavily it leaks like a sieve.

"Last winter the water ran straight through the roof into the trauma care department," says a tall Canadian OR nurse.

"If the roof already struggles to stop rain from coming in, we can only hope a 107mm-missile never lands on top of it," I respond.

As I look at the ceiling, I realise once again I just said those words out loud. I direct my gaze to the floor rather than the ceiling. No one seems to have heard what I said or wants to make a big deal about it.

We continue our extensive tour of the hospital. Our tour guide explains in detail all we need to know about the capacities the hospital has to provide its patients with the best possible care.

The area that the Role 3 hospital is responsible for is enormous. Care is provided to more than 18,000 personnel at the camp as well as to tens of thousands of coalition troops in southern Afghanistan. It also offers life and limb saving care to the Afghan troops and police force.

A wide range of care is offered within the complex of the plywood hovel and the cluster of tents and containers. It varies from help to those with a common cold to specialist care for victims of gunfights and roadside bombs.

Civilian casualties won't usually come to the hospital, unless they are the result of direct combat related violence. When they are a victim of a targeted attack, we will help them and perform surgery. We will also assist the local Afghan Mirwais hospital when it can't handle the stream of injured patients and will help out if there is a lack of medical expertise in Mirwais to perform certain procedures. Only if we have the capacity, we take on some of the local hospital's patients.

Then there are other patients who are a bit of a grey area. My Canadian colleague tells us that Afghan children also end up on our hospital's operating table, even when their injuries aren't combat related. This is a way of winning hearts and minds.

〜

The hospital has access to a *trauma care department,* the *emergency room* (ER) for airlifted patients. Nine patients can be taken in and stabilised at the same time. The surgical capacity consists of two operating rooms. One of these is mainly equipped to deal with orthopaedic procedures, whilst the other one is more tailored to general surgery. The ward can accommodate a maximum of ten patients and the ICU, *Intensive Care Unit*, has four beds. There also are auxiliary departments, like an X-ray department including a CT-scanner, a laboratory, a blood bank, a dental department, physiotherapy and family medicine.

"Well, it's not actually that big here, is it? Really, there are only ten hospital beds," I ask my Canadian colleague whilst I look at him inquisitively.

He smiles from ear to ear and agrees. "We're often full. If that's the case, there is the possibility to, in case of an emergency, divert to a big tent behind the hospital. That's where we can hold another 20 patients. These would be the ones who, for example, are able to walk and need less intensive care."

The policy at the hospital is that wounded members of the coalition forces are stabilised and will only undergo vital, urgent surgery. Then it is a matter of evacuating them without delay to a higher level of care, so that they can be taken care of under more ideal circumstances.

It is different for Afghan forces, police and civilians. They are brought to our Role 3 hospital and their treatment plan is then aimed at making sure they will leave the hospital as soon as possible, without needing any more care.

≈

Our Canadian colleague tells us that patients are not the only Afghans we will encounter in the hospital. Indeed, during our deployment we meet a trio of Afghan men that seems to be present

24 hours a day. Day in, day out they clean the hospital armed with a mop stick and a cleaning trolley. Immediately after they have finished cleaning the final room, they start at the beginning again. These fanatical cleaners also function as contracted interpreters. They are indispensable, because they enable us to have some communication with the Afghan patients. They are employed by ISAF, the *International Security Assistance Force*. According to Afghan standards they earn a good salary.

I wonder about the background of these ever-smiling interpreters. Apparently, they were lucky enough to have access to some education. Did they belong to the *upper classes* before the fighting started? I assume they were lawyers or teachers. Shouldn't they stand up and be involved in the future of their country? Perhaps, one day, if they are lucky, they receive a green card to build a new life for themselves and flee their homeland. That might be a wonderful prospect for the interpreter, but isn't it a massive loss for the country?

I don't want to dwell on this too long. I am here to contribute to the care of individual patients. I am going to 'perform my trick' by being there for the victims and by helping to save lives.

In a few months I will go back to my lovely home. Back to my loving wife and children.

WARMING-UP

"Drink, drink, drink, and every time you take a piss you have to check to make sure it doesn't look like dark tea. And if it does? You've guessed it right: drink some more." This is what we are told to do to deal with the heat. It is no mean feat to drink an extra eight to nine litres per day, but it is vital we do so. During summer, temperatures in this region easily reach more than 50 °C in the shade. These are conditions that we are not used to, and they need to be dealt with properly.

We are briefed about a programme that focuses on making sure troops that have just arrived at the camp get accustomed to the climate as quickly as possible. Besides drinking fluids, other practical points with regards to the goings on at the camp are discussed.

At the end of the briefing we hear that our surgical team is excluded from the adaptation programme and that we will have to find our own ways to adapt to the climate.

This exclusion confirms to me that I am part of a club of outsiders. We are a team of people pieced together from a hospital that has now been added to a bigger unit. In this desert we will carry out our highly specialised task, detached from everyone and everything. We will, once our time is up, leave theatre in the same solitary and anonymous way as we arrived. It makes me feel inferior and like I don't belong.

As a small team of individuals, we will be under command of TFU-3, *Task Force Uruzgan*. The majority of the unit will be deployed to Tarin Kowt or Deh Rawod in the Uruzgan province. We, however, are deployed to the airfield of Kandahar in the province with the same name.

From the moment we started our preparations, I felt that our team and the command unit never really had a connection and this feeling would only grow over time. Where the whole unit already collaborated during preparation for the deployment, we only became part of it at the last moment. The surgical team is like the appendix of the unit. It is there, but it is not clear what use it has and above all it shouldn't be causing any trouble.

Aren't we important enough to take part in the programme that prepares us for the heat too? We are also casually told that it is not sure our team will be flown home via Crete after the deployment for the decompression days. It had already been mentioned to us during our preparations, but it still feels as if we are inferior.

I actually feel some resentment. Are double standards applied here? I wonder why? Is it negligence on behalf of our medical command unit at home? Have they not signed us up, or do they think we don't need it? Do they simply assume we are not going to be that busy? Or do I worry too much about it and should I just wait and see what happens?

As a final insult we hear we won't be stationed in the Dutch section of the camp for much longer. We are going to be transferred to the Canadian camp, nearly half a mile away.

"All in the name of togetherness," I once again think out loud. My words are dripping with sarcasm.

We have familiarised ourselves with all procedures and practices over the last two days. The team we are due to relieve will be heading home shortly, and from that day onwards we will be on our own.

The friendly and very tall Canadian nurse, who has been showing us around and has taught us all the ins and outs, chats about the ups and downs of the hospital. We listen closely to him. Recently, it hasn't been that busy looking at the number of victims that have been brought in. The variety and severity of the injuries have made a huge impression on him though. He tells us that it is not only the nature of injuries that has contributed to the impact the war has made on him. The 'them and us feeling' that is prevalent also plays a part. He describes how injured coalition colleagues have made a far more lasting impression on him than a Taliban fighter has done.

"Some days it is as if you are on an emotional roller-coaster," he continues calmly. "Performing surgery in these circumstances has two sides. What I have experienced here is the highest achievable from a professional point of view, and on an emotional level it is top sport." He describes the creativity that is needed during operations and he talks a lot about thinking and working *out of the box*, teamwork and the initiatives that are necessary to be able to do as much possible for patients. He presents all of this as a fabulous marketing campaign, but behind his smile I can see he has experienced a lot.

It is clear to me that this job can be challenging. All possible injuries have to be treated, but there is only a limited number of specialists and surgical personnel available: two general surgeons, two orthopaedic surgeons, a maxillofacial surgeon and a vascular surgeon. Together, we will treat every conceivable trauma.

There are two surgical teams and two operating rooms. In the worst-case scenario, when it is extremely busy, both teams will be working in both ORs simultaneously. During these moments there is no back-up and there is no night shift that comes in at the end of the day like at home. We continue to work till we have finished surgery on our last patient.

"A 24-hour shift for the Dutch, followed by 24 hours for the Canadian team. If needed, you will be called back in, for example when more than one patient is brought in," he tells us. "But that doesn't happen very often."

He was wrong.

~

Looking around the emergency room of the hospital, I remember a documentary about a field hospital during the war in Iraq that I saw prior to my deployment. There were lots of casualties, some with two or more severed limbs and that footage left a lasting impression. I hope we will be spared this, though I fully realise we will probably experience it, given the amount of IED attacks that are taking place. Severely injured soldiers from the coalition forces but also children will end up on our operating tables, and when that happens we will be ready to help them survive.

Just a few days ago, three Canadian soldiers lost their lives in an attack and the shock can still be felt around the base and in the hospital. It has damaged the feeling of togetherness. The casualties were flown home yesterday, after a farewell ceremony.

When members of the coalition forces have died, a *ramp ceremony* is organised. During such a ceremony hundreds of troops stand to attention on the platform with a guard of honour made up of colleagues. One-by-one the coffins are carried on the shoulders of their comrades to the plane that will take them home one last time. We would have to go through many of these ceremonies and the first one would happen quicker than I could have imagined.

~

A new patient has just been admitted to the hospital. I observe from an appropriate distance, take it all in and look at how everything functions. Everybody in the ER is concentrating and working efficiently. Their efficiency betrays that they have been working together for quite some time. A textbook example of international collaboration is happening right before my eyes. Doctors and nurses from Canada, the USA, the UK, New Zealand and the Netherlands collaborate like a well-oiled machine and as one team they work on the patient whose life is at stake.

They work in full force to stabilise him. Vital stats are called out and noted down, IVs and central lines are inserted, and an extensive physical examination is performed. The man isn't responsive; he is on life support. I can't help but look past everyone and count the patient's limbs. He still has all four.

The Afghan soldier, who lies motionless on the stretcher, suffers from a severe head trauma. Sarcastically I think that it looks like he has tried to stop something big with his head. He obviously failed as his entire forehead has been pushed in by almost an inch.

A little later the CT-scan images are displayed on a screen. I have a quick look at them over the surgeon's shoulder and catch some of the doctors having a chat amongst themselves. It is not looking good for the patient, this is a so-called *dead man walking*. He is already dead, he just doesn't know it yet. I turn around and walk away.

That night I ring the home front. "Hi love, everything's alright here. The hospital seems to be a good place to work. It does look a bit rustic. Well, that's an understatement. It's super rustic, but I'll find my feet. I'll be fine here."

I tell my wife that I saw the first patient injured because of military violence today. I decide not to mention that the injuries were so profound that he was dying there and then.

Then I speak to my sons and ask them if they are being good and only take one sweet each out of the jar every day.

"I miss you, boys. Daddy loves you."

After the phone call I walk back to my tent. Whilst I am sitting on my bed I drink another bottle of water. I have actually lost count. I think about the man with the head injury for a minute. The percentage of deaths in this hospital is probably higher than in a regular hospital with ideal circumstances. It comes with the territory, as a war is raging in this country ruled by local tribes and drug dealers. The central government doesn't seem to have any influence whatsoever. Why would we think we can make a difference here at all? I have the feeling that the only difference I will be able to make, is limited to helping the injured individual who ends up on our operating table. This is the image I try and hold on to, and I try to prevent that I am overcome by a feeling of utter futility already.

A cacophony of sounds resonates through the hospital. The noise of drilling and sawing by workmen drowns out the beeping of the monitors in the emergency room.

The hospital's interior can change day by day. A new crew of workmen arrived a few days ago. Armed with sheets of plywood and beams they are building another new wing to the cabin. There are several builders at work in the hospital every single day. It is being developed and changed all the time and it is never completely sure if a certain wall or area will still be there the next day.

In the midst of all this noise the maxillofacial surgeon is concentrating on the computer screen. I look at the screen too and see an X-ray of the face of the patient who has just been brought in.

"Unbelievable, another face that has been shot to pieces. This is going to be some job."

I do my best to hear him over all the construction sounds. The injury is so severe that this patient has to go into surgery straight away. When he comes past on the stretcher, I see the devastation that is his face. It sends shivers down my spine.

Moments later he is on the operating table. The surgeon has to perform a *tracheostomy*, which means putting a breathing tube through his throat. Inserting a tube through the mouth was simply not possible anymore. Where his mouth used to be is now a gaping hole, the result of a gunshot. A bullet must have entered his face through the left cheek, and must have exited through the right jaw where there was once a chin. His jaw on the left side is still reasonably intact, with just a small bullet hole visible. The bullet transformed both mouth and jaw into one gaping, bloody mass. The patient's tongue has been severely damaged. His right cheek is now only connected to the mandibular by a few fibres and the part of the jawbone between the mandibular angle and the right-hand side of the chin is completely gone. This man will be lucky to ever talk, eat and drink normally again. At home, an injury like this would, under ideal circumstances, require a lengthy period of rehabilitation. In this country that is impossible. He will eventually be discharged from our hospital or transferred to a local civilian hospital after which he will have to fend for himself.

While the patient is being prepared for surgery, I wonder if it is at all possible for someone who is so seriously injured to live independently. People have to literally fight to survive here. Only the strongest will make it and this man will have no one to rely on but himself. A dreadful prospect.

At the same time though, my professional ego figures this will be a really interesting surgery. It is going to take a good few hours and we will have to pull out all the stops to help the patient get through it. After watching and assisting for some time I walk out of theatre and grab a fresh bottle of water.

War surgery already impresses me. The patients who come to this hospital, straight from where the damage is done, and their injuries affect me whether I want them to or not. It is extraordinary that we are dealing with such complicated issues and that we work with the little means we have available. We have to make the best of what we got. I just hope we have got enough.

When I am halfway through my bottle of water, my Canadian colleague comes looking for us and asks us to immediately get to work in the second operating room. An injured American soldier arrived only a moment ago. It will be my first surgery of many.

~

Pain is etched on the young man's face. He seems to be hyper alert and his bright blue eyes search for ours. His left hand supports his right wrist, and he groans when we help him onto the operating table. The X-ray shows a fracture in the lower arm. This Role 3 hospital will be the end station of his deployment. After surgery he will be flown to Germany for follow-up treatment. His fracture will first need to be stabilised by us with an Ex-Fix, an external fixator.

An external fixator is nothing more than a temporary way to stabilise a fracture, outside of the body. Holes are drilled in the unaffected bone on either side of the fracture. Special pins are then screwed in the holes. Next, metal or synthetic rods are attached to these pins which secure everything. A special bull joint between the rod and the pins ensures the fracture can be placed in the correct anatomical position after which it is set in place.

"I'm such an asshole! I've abandoned my mates," the soldier moans on the operating table. He is talking to no one in particular. "The Taliban have been trying for months to kill or injure me and my buddies. They haven't succeeded. Today, I don't pay attention for two seconds and I trip. I hear a snapping noise and I know something's wrong. How stupid can you be?"

I am positioned at the head end of the operating table next to the patient. He briefly glances at the floor, sees my big yellow Dutch wooden shoes and starts to grin. "Dude, really?" He grins and then, with renewed vigour, he continues to moan about himself and the rest of Afghanistan.

"Go and sleep, mate. Find yourself a nice dream. We're going to take good care of you. Sleep tight." I say this to all patients just before we send them off to sleep, also to the ones for whom these will be the last words they will ever hear.

His swearing and moaning gets quieter and becomes more and more disjointed as the anaesthetist resolutely empties the syringe into the bloodstream of this unfortunate soldier. We managed to stabilise the fracture. My colleague Linda assists the surgeon during the procedure, whilst I am the circulating nurse, in charge of the equipment and supplies.

After the surgery I sit in the shade behind the hospital and smoke a cigarette. I inhale deeply and exhale a big cloud of smoke. We just performed surgery on our first patient. I note it down in a few short sentences on an empty page of my little diary. I would continue to do this during my entire stay in Afghanistan.

A LOGISTICAL LABYRINTH

It has only been a few days since I set foot in Afghanistan. On my first day the camp was plagued by an enormous rain shower. In a short space of time the entire base transformed from a dry moon-like landscape to something resembling a typical Dutch autumnal scene. After that day, the sun appeared and the temperature quickly rose to an enormous height.

The heat is only bearable early in the morning, which is when I go running. When I step outside in my running gear at half past five in the morning and walk into the fresh air I get goosebumps or even shiver a bit. At this time the thermometer indicates a 'cool' 28 degrees Celsius. Around midday though the temperature rises to around 45 degrees Celsius, in the shade.

It is a lot more pleasant in the hospital. In every room, including the operating rooms, there are one or more air conditioners, ensuring the temperature is a constant 24 degrees Celsius. That is quite comfortable for a working environment.

We work long days in the relative coolness of the operating room. Every time we go outside, either to smoke a cigarette or to take away amputated limbs or other medical waste, it feels like we are being slapped in the face. I would never really get used to the high outdoor temperatures.

Other than my way around the hospital I have also managed to get to know my way around the rest of the huge base by now. There is a big open space in the centre, which is used as a sports field. This area is surrounded by a wooden boardwalk, with along it several containers housing little shops. There are also trailers for big chains like Burger King, Pizza Hut and Subway. It is weird to see a Burger King in the middle of the desert of war-torn Afghanistan. Even though I had planned to go and have a look I still haven't done that.

~

The fluorescent lighting behind the operating rooms is not quite sufficient to light up the whole corridor. On both sides there are heavy metal shelves full of sterile instrument sets and it is only just wide enough to be able to walk past each other. The shelves are fully covered by curtains, which are there to keep the packed sets free from dust.

The fine dust particles, which penetrate absolutely everything, find their way around the whole hospital. This is because the 'plywood shed' has not been designed to be dust free and also because the air-conditioning is always on, injecting Afghan dust into the operating rooms and the rest of the hospital.

The corridor, which is too narrow and dark, is the heart of the hospital's storage. This is where nearly all of the materials that are used during surgery are stored; varying from advanced drilling and sawing equipment to dressings to take care of the most gruesome wounds.

"Make sure that you walk along this corridor hundreds of times and look to your left and right each time you do so. Try to memorise

37

where everything is, because there is no logic to it whatsoever," I hear someone say.

The side that is closest to the operating theatres stores all the instrument sets, the individual instruments and also the implants like screws, plates and intramedullary rods. These all seem to be stored in a reasonably logical way, as opposed to the other sterile resources.

"Erik, can you quickly fetch some stump dressings?" Linda asks.

This marks the start of a new search for me. I am sure I found this specific bandage before, but where? Sighing, I walk up and down the corridor. I moan about the shabby lighting and curse the storage, where nothing is where it should be. There is not one labelled shelf. It is like looking for a needle in a haystack.

It happens frequently that several people have to search for one particular emergency set. Stock management doesn't exist here, even though searching is sometimes literally a matter of life or death.

In the operating room we often have to make do because of the lack of space. Surgical lights are placed at such a height that anyone of average height is doomed to constantly hit their heads. Each and every time I turn around to get another instrument to pass to the surgeon, I bump into the light. Invariably, this is accompanied by an unmistakably blunt expletive. At the end of our deployment our Canadian colleagues would be able to rant and swear in Dutch fluently.

After a bit of a hunt, I find the necessary dressings. They are well hidden behind a pile of urinary catheters. "That makes sense," I groan, as I grab the box of dressings and place it prominently in front of the catheters. Whoever is going to be looking for a catheter will now have trouble finding it.

When I walk back into the operating room, I nearly trip over a red rubbish bag placed at the entrance. The amputated arm of the Afghan soldier on our operating table is in the red bag. I only just manage to keep myself upright. Everyone in the room starts to laugh. Tripping over my own feet I triumphantly hold the stump bandage up in the air.

"Brilliant time, Erik. That could well be a new record."

~

The young American soldier with the broken arm we operated on earlier today, is in a bed on the ward. He is wide awake and is looking at his arm which is all wrapped up in white, spotless bandages. The contraption that holds the fracture in place sticks out from under all the dressings. The guy seems lost in thought as I walk past his bed.

The external fixator procedure is a standard procedure for wounded ISAF colleagues. There are huge supplies of this sort of material in storage. For our Afghan patients we have other supplies ready and waiting. Their treatment is fully focused on recovering in the shortest possible timeframe. They would therefore hardly ever get an external fixator, because that means he would have to come back for follow-up surgery. Instead, they would have an intramedullary rod for a leg or arm fracture; a metal pin which is placed in the medullary cavity of the bone of, for example, the upper or lower leg. This pin is fastened with screws and stabilises the fracture, so it won't need any more treatment.

The patient would be discharged from hospital relatively quickly after which they would recover in their own surroundings. This is of course good for the patient, but it also helps the intake capacity of the hospital. Everything is geared towards discharging patients from the hospital as quickly as is medically justified. There is only a limited number of hospital beds which are all desperately needed.

Pins and screws in all shapes and sizes are stored in the corridor behind the theaters. Placing these intramedullary rods would become a frequent procedure. At the end of our deployment we would almost be able to perform this procedure with our eyes closed.

The victim on the stretcher at the ER is unsettled. A non-stop deluge of unintelligible Afghan words comes out of his mouth, as if he is singing or praying. His head moves violently from left to right and he looks around wildly.

The young man is extremely tense and seems to want to get up constantly. He won't be able to. His clothes have been cut open and are piled up under the stretcher on the blood-covered floor. His legs are severely injured with holes blown into them in multiple places. These holes seem to be the result of an explosion. This man will have to forget about walking independently for the time being.

His right arm is seriously damaged too. Just above a huge, gaping wound is a tightened tourniquet, ensuring the bleeding has now stopped. The most noteworthy aspect of the patient's arms isn't the wound or the compression bandage though. It is the fact that they are tied together; he appears to be handcuffed. A wide tie-wrap is tightly wrapped around his wrists.

The attending interpreter who, earlier today, was busy mopping the floors, is now wearing a surgical mask and massive, jet-black sunglasses that cover nearly his entire face. He talks to the injured man incessantly. If his goal is to calm the patient, it looks like he is failing.

It suddenly dawns on me that this patient is a captured suspect. This young, bearded guy is handcuffed on the stretcher, preventing him from doing us harm, and the interpreter, employed by the coalition forces, has made sure he cannot be recognised.

Later, he would tell me that people known to be connected to ISAF have been tortured and killed by insurgents before. Sometimes the helpful man's complete family is murdered as a warning to him and his fellow villagers. Since knowing this, my respect has grown for these interpreters who risk their own lives, and that of their families, to devote themselves to the coalition troops.

Even though this handcuffed talib is everyone's enemy in the hospital, first and foremost he is a patient now, and is entitled to the same support any other injured person gets. We are the ones who will give him that support. While I stand at the foot end of the stretcher I observe how my colleagues from the emergency room work on him. They help the man to sit up so they can listen to his heart and lungs with a stethoscope.

Suddenly he looks at me and in his eyes I see pure hate. For a split second I want to look away, but I decide not to. I stare back at him and show no emotions at all.

The second patient is significantly calmer. All we hear from him are continuous groans. His face is heavily wounded. Where his bottom left jaw used to be, is nothing more than a bloody mass. The rest of his face is caked in dried blood, dirt and dust. The X-rays show that what is left of his jaw is completely shattered. This will be a task for the maxillofacial surgeon and it definitely won't be an easy one.

The impact of being a war victim unfolds right before my eyes. This is not simply a broken jaw. This is a jaw that, for the most part, has been destroyed by violence. A fragment hit this policeman's face and obliterated everything in its path. Was this explosion caused by the talib who is here too?

I wonder if this man will ever be able to function properly again. This trauma isn't remedied by just reconstructing his jaw. His tongue is so severely damaged that the majority of it will have to be removed. This young police officer will need to learn how to speak all over again.

I stick around for the surgery that is performed by the Canadian team. Sweat is pouring down the face of the maxillofacial surgeon. After some intense hours of surgery the mandibular has been reconstructed. It will remain to be seen whether it is going to be functional.

After the operation I have a short chat with the surgeon. He warmly welcomes us as the new team and explains that this patient will have more surgeries. The reconstructed jaw will be closely monitored. He also tells me that it is normal practice in this hospital to perform numerous surgeries on the same patient. He hasn't had that many patients on the operating table during his deployment, but in the same breath he mentions that nearly every patient will come back for additional surgery.

"There's always something to do here," he grins.

~

We would perform lots of maxillofacial surgery and operate on many patients whose faces were destroyed. All of those made a lasting impact on me. I often wondered whether the reconstructions would actually deliver the desired results.

After these sorts of procedures, I would often retreat to my usual spot behind the hospital, smoking one cigarette after another, whilst my doubt about our care continued to grow. From a medical-technical point of view we would deliver a masterpiece more than once, but at the same time I would be unsure what quality of life we would offer our patients.

"Another poor guy who will never be able to nonchalantly hang a cigarette from the corner of his mouth again. He might never talk again," I say out loud, to no-one in particular.

"Fucking war."

KEEPING UP APPEARANCES

I throw cloth after cloth in the rubbish bag. They are all impregnated with a strong disinfectant. Each of them has changed from spotless white to dull grey. We have been cleaning both operating rooms for over an hour. Loud music sounds through the whole of the department and Linda and I are singing along as loudly as possible. Once in a while a nurse pops his head around the door and looks at us in bewilderment. When that happens both Linda and I stop in our tracks for a moment to wave like a bunch of fools at our audience, resulting in the nurse to quickly walk away, with a smile on the face.

Cleaning the department is a daily ritual. Each morning when we arrive at the hospital, every single square inch of the ORs is covered in a thin layer of fine dust. It regularly manages to jam the air-conditioning system, quickly resulting in unbearably hot operating rooms. Almost daily I am amazed that we are here in the middle of the desert and when we see dust and dirt, we simply wipe it away after which we put the most severely wounded patients on the operating table. There isn't even an adequate air treatment system, inconceivable in the hospital at home where a constant stream of clean air has to be guaranteed, and the OR has to be spotless before any surgical procedures can be performed.

Interestingly enough, we would hardly come across any postoperative infections. I don't know if this is because people here have a better immune system resulting in less infections or because we are simply too frantic about hygiene at home.

~

"I've caught it, Linda!"

I hear a short and sharp crunching sound under my clog.

"What was it?" she asks.

I tell her it was a massive, black beetle.

She walks over to the whiteboard on the wall of the operating room and adds a new line in the column called beetles. It is the third one this week to lose its life in our OR.

We normally use the whiteboard to keep track of the amount of sterile gauzes needed during surgery, so that we can check if all of them are indeed removed from the patient's body at the end of the procedure. We have slightly modified the use of the board.

Next to the columns for the gauzes are now some extra ones to list the insects most regularly found in this operating room. The bodycount of insects killed by us is noted down behind each different type.

At home, newspapers often dedicate whole articles to the news that a hospital is temporarily closed because of the presence of mosquitoes or flies, yet here they are regular visitors and no one seems to worry too much about them. We enthusiastically hunt these intruders down and the tally is growing steadily. With great determination we try to ambush and then eliminate as many beetles, mosquitoes, flies, spiders and other unwelcome guests as possible. The full bodyweight of a huge scrub nurse in large, yellow Dutch wooden shoes works wonders. Intruders with even the thickest of armours cannot withstand this brute force. It is a welcome distraction from the daily grind of cleaning, preparing, stocking and tidying the operating rooms.

~

It takes a couple of seconds before I realise that the insistent beeping I hear actually comes from my pocket. I am alert and on edge as soon as I comprehend what it is. It is the hospital's beeper, which indicates through a code on the screen that we have to return immediately.

Multiple victims are en route to the hospital. I get up from the large picnic table. Moments ago, I treated myself to a fresh cup of coffee and slightly disappointed, I glance one last time at my plastic cup with steaming hot coffee. Then I get rid of the last bit of my cigarette and start to walk to the hospital.

When I arrive, there are lots of people preparing for what is to come. There is a large notice board in a central position on the wall. This is where, bit by bit, all the available information is noted down about the injured that are due to come in and about those who have already been brought in.

The scribbled down words on the board tell us that we can expect two wounded Afghan police officers, who have been hit by an explosion. The only extra information we receive is that both are alive and have numerous blast wounds. The notice board in the corridor doesn't give any guarantees though.

Every time it remains to be seen if what is noted down for us will actually come in. If something is written on the board, it means at best that wounded people are on their way. The number of patients and the nature of their injuries are usually stated, but it is 'free to interpretation.' One particular time three heavily wounded soldiers were supposed to be on their way, whereas one child was brought in who wasn't quite ten years old yet. Clearly a bad connection somewhere.

Whilst I look at the board I notice that someone is standing behind me. It is the American chaplain. We have a short, animated conversation. He appears to be cheerful, but I can see that he has been at this hospital for quite some time. The look in his eyes betrays that he has seen and experienced more than enough.

I wonder if I will have the same look in my eyes in a couple of weeks. I hope not. I have only been here for a short while, but I already know that distressing injuries pass through the hospital and that the days can be tough, virtually unbearable even. At present it is all manageable though and I hope it stays that way.

Slowly the rest of the team arrives. We check if the operating room is ready to go and once we have assured ourselves of this, all we can do is wait for the patients that will be brought in. The ER, in the meantime, is a hive of activity. Key personnel wear different coloured hats signifying what their roles are. We stay in the background.

The scene that unfolds right before my eyes is like a TV programme, but with one big difference. In this hospital nothing is dramatised and the patients actually can succumb to their injuries. There is no director who shouts 'cut', when a take isn't quite to his liking.

The atmosphere changes, as soon as the stretchers enter the hospital and the tension that could be felt a short while ago changes into efficiency, while the trauma department transforms into a well-organised anthill.

"Trauma 1! Put him in Trauma 1!" a superior shouts when the first stretcher is wheeled in. It is attached to a mobile base. The casualty is motionless. Straddling him on the stretcher is an American medic who is performing CPR on him.

"Nearly thirty minutes now, with intervals," he responds to the question of how long he has been doing this for. Sweat runs down his cheeks from under his aircrew helmet and drips onto the wounded Afghan policeman. This youthful looking casualty is as white as a sheet. He is quickly taken to the trauma bay, immediately opposite our operating theatre, where we are ready and waiting.

An ER colleague takes over the resuscitation from the flight nurse, who was in the helicopter with the injured man. He takes off his helmet, wipes his face and stretches. He looks pained and for a moment he watches the team fight for the life of this young police officer. Then he turns around, shakes his head and walks back to the helicopter, which is still waiting for him.

We are still waiting patiently until someone shouts to let us know we can start work. It is an awful feeling to just have to watch without being able to do anything.

"How long have we been resuscitating for?" the anaesthetist asks.

"Just over forty-two minutes," is the reply.

We have taken all the steps as per the protocol and are going to try one last time." Once again, several vials of medication are intravenously administered to the patient. Everyone looks at the monitor that displays the patient's vital stats. Nothing changes on the screen at all.

"Does anyone have any ideas on how we can turn this around?"

It stays eerily quiet. What follows is a brief command to stop resuscitating.

"Time of death: 1.56pm."

∾

The second casualty is taken to another bay. The ER team immediately tries to stabilise him. His arm is badly damaged. He will undergo a few additional examinations after which he will go into surgery straight away.

After we have double-checked that the OR is set for the patient with the destroyed arm, I step out of the hospital, light a cigarette and think about the fact that we just lost our surgical patient before we were even able to do anything for him at all.

I watched the death of a young policeman, without being able to lend a hand. When I glance at the whiteboard a few moments later, I notice that this patient has been crossed out. Immediately after his patient number there is now a bold cross, and the time of death. Statistically this is not a good start. I hope this won't be a trend.

~

"Erik, let's go."

I throw away the last bit of my umpteenth cigarette and with big steps I walk back inside. In passing, I grab a dry scrub top from the pile, put it on and make my way to the OR, just as the patient is wheeled in.

The damage to the arm is impressive. Because of the explosion and the released pressure accompanying the blast, the flying shards and debris have made a hole in the left arm of three by nearly five inches. In a split second, the explosion changed all underlying structures into a mushy soup. On the X-rays we can see that both bones in the lower arm have been totally destroyed and we also see lots of small, bright white spots everywhere.

"Those spots are pieces of foreign material," the surgeon says. They are shard fragments.

When I see the X-rays, I suspect this arm is lost and I don't expect us to be able to save it. We would have to amputate.

The protocol for amputated limbs of Afghan patients is that the limb is packed in a double red rubbish bag. We attach a label to it with the relevant patient number and it is then taken to a huge, chilled container outside of the hospital. This is where the limb is stored until the patient is discharged. It then gets passed on to the patient or their family. I tell myself that it is all part of their culture.

I check if there are any red bags in the operating room. They are, however, not needed quite yet as the goal is to try and save the arm at all costs. The patient on our table is a close relative of a local dignitary and therefore amputating is not an option at the moment. First, all other possibilities need to be completely exhausted.

We start the time-consuming tasks of not only reconstructing both bones in the lower arm, but also of extensive vascular surgery. We will have to mend the affected muscles and nerves as best as we can.

The police officer, who descends from an upper-class family, has a full head of greying hair. I wonder if the attack was aimed at him specifically? He has wounds all over his body from the debris that was flying around and his skin has a dull grey colour because of the dust. Where there is no dust, there are little holes, soot and dried-up, clotted blood on his body.

Whilst my colleague, dressed in sterile clothing, makes sure all the instruments and supplies are ready for the operation, I focus on preparing the patient. I clean the parts of his body that will be operated on after which I disinfect his whole arm. As soon as that is done, I cover it with sterile surgical drapes.

"Just move a tiny bit, Erik and turn the arm towards me for a sec. Thanks, and another one close up. Nice, nice, nice!"

To the left and right of me I hear the clicking of cameras, whilst I am wrapping up the arm. Before we can start surgery, some people in the operating room want to take pictures at all angles. After a while I feel that, rather than working to actually save the injured man's limb, I am posing with a damaged arm in my hands. Slowly but surely I get annoyed.

"If you're so desperate for a picture, why don't you ask him for some, the one with the big camera. He has more than enough pictures to share!" I snap, while I keep on working.

As soon as I finish covering up the patient and checking that everything is set for surgery, I sit down near my colleague, so that she can ask me for extra supplies when needed.

The procedure finally starts and one by one the paparazzi leave the room. Everyone concentrates on what needs to be done: saving an arm.

I observe for a while. The entire arm is opened up on both the in- and outside and all underlying structures are restored, as far as possible. It quickly becomes clear that the end goal is a functional arm. That is why this patient will have to come back for a second operation in a couple of weeks.

"I don't think it's right that those pictures had be taken first, when the guy's arm needed our attention," Linda says.

I agree, not knowing it would get far worse. Pictures would have to be taken of every single detail of every patient, unless there was simply no time for photographers to be running around, because we would be doing what we were actually there for: saving lives.

After several hours the limb is saved, for the time being at least. More operations would have to follow to give this patient a functioning arm. He would take up one of the beds for quite some time and then return for a bone graft. This is where part of the fibula would be taken to be implanted in the affected arm. During this procedure we would also perform a skin graft. This would close up the large, gaping hole in his arm.

I wonder if the same choice would have been made for an Afghan soldier from a different walk of life. Would we have pulled out all the stops to save his arm? I don't dare to ask that question. I have no reason to believe that this is what has happened, but I get the feeling that I have just experienced a mild form of class justice. It looks like we have had to try a bit harder, only because this patient is more highly regarded than others. It continues to be a feeling I don't dare to share with others.

Once the patient has woken up, we take him to the one and only single room in this hospital. This is the room that is normally used to take care of hospitalised detainees. The man will be looked after in this private room until he is sufficiently recovered to undergo additional surgery. The best-case scenario is that this operation should ensure that he will be able to use his arm better. The worst-case scenario is that his lower arm will still be amputated after all.

After the long surgery, we sit down together with some colleagues to drink a cup of coffee and discuss the operation. It doesn't take long until we place our first bets on the next surgery and whether or not we will be able to save the patient's arm.

The sun has set by the time I leave hospital. I wander over to the Dutch camp with Linda. I badly need a cup of coffee that actually tastes like coffee.

I meet a couple of guys who are in transit to Deh Rawod. They will leave the base daily to be in great danger. I tell them that I have a lot of respect for them, but they immediately turn the conversation around to tell us how much respect they have for the work we do. Assisting to save life and limbs captures their imagination.

"Let's make a deal not to meet each other whilst you're on shift," says the bearded infantryman who has been quiet up to this point, as he looks around whilst walking off. Sheer determination glistens in his eyes.

"We better not. Wear a helmet!" I grin sheepishly.

He gives me a thumbs-up. "Deal."

I rehearsed the phone call I am about to have a couple of times in my head. "I have ended up in such a shithole. A young guy was brought in today and we weren't able to help him at all. The last bit of life left his body and all I could do was watch it happen. I realise after these first couple of days that I am in the middle of a war zone. I do not feel safe, despite the relative protection of this huge, heavily guarded base. We're in the fucking middle of Taliban country, thank goodness we haven't been shot at yet."

This is what I had planned to say to my wife, but as soon as she answers the phone and I hear the happiness in her voice, I decide against it. "Everything is going well here, sweetheart. Work was good. We had such an interesting case on the operating table today, which kept us busy for a while. The holiday brochures were telling the truth, you know. It is definitely a trip with guaranteed sun. How are the kids? Give them a big kiss from me. I'm happy to hear your voice. I'll try and ring again tomorrow!" I have started to keep up appearances.

I can't let go off the image of my colleague covered in sweat, pushing down on the chest of that guy who was way too young to die. A man, who followed his dream of joining the police force to help stabilise his country, has died. He was mowed down because of what he stood for and we haven't been able to help him. We walk away from him to keep doing what we are doing for another patient, who is someone of a higher rank. A patient for whom we pull out all the stops to successfully save his arm.

Would the same thing have happened if the young guy who is in the mortuary now had that same injury? Or would we have immediately amputated his arm?

I am not sure if I understand it all. Is there not a golden rule which states that all patients have to be treated equally, without exception? It feels like the opposite has happened today. It took place right before my eyes and I cooperated with it.

I don't want to think about it. Just let me get on with what I came for and what I am good at. Assisting surgeons. Assisting, yes. Passing cutlery, yes. Offering the best possible patient care, yes absolutely, that is what I am here for and what I am good at. But where does good patient care stop and does it actually become 'making it up as we go along'? I don't know, but this will probably happen more often.

～

For quite some time now and only a dozen miles away from the airport, a small Canadian unit has been under fire. A large group of militants has ambushed and attacked the ISAF soldiers with small calibre firearms and *rocket-propelled grenades* (RPGs), which are shoulder-launched anti-tank weapons.

Reinforcements of the Afghan army have become involved to extract the Canadian unit, and the air support out of Kandahar Airfield that has been requested, is on its way. Two heavily-armed F-16 Fighting Falcons have just taken off to bring relief to the Canadians. The fight has been going on for several hours and multiple casualties have been reported.

The Canadians are extracted after an intense firefight lasting more than three hours. The hostile militants retreat when reinforcement and air support arrive. There are fatalities and casualties for both ISAF and the militants.

～

It is really early in the morning. The sun has just started to rise and it promises to be another sweltering day.

The beeper sounds before breakfast is even finished. I was hoping for a rest day. That is not going to happen again.

I swear loudly as I put on my fatigues. I grab a bottle of water from a pallet and make my way to the hospital.

The report tells us we are dealing with masscal, *massive casualties*. This means multiple casualties will be brought in at the same time. It is quite a flexible concept though. Whenever we receive the masscal message, the question is what is really going to be coming in. Will it be two or twenty? Are we actually going to be needed or will they all be dead before they even arrive? That last scenario would happen sooner rather than later and would prove to be a huge blow for all of us.

In case of masscal, everyone who has a post within Role 3 is beeped at the same time. This means that the cosy wooden shed quickly transforms into a crowded cabin where everyone is preparing for the arrival of casualties.

On the whiteboard next to the operating theatre we read that five casualties are on their way. A Canadian soldier and two enemy fighters have been injured. Their injuries consist of shrapnel trauma and bullet wounds.

There are also two more soldiers on their way, both from the Afghan army and with the VSA status, *vital signs absent*.

When we receive the news that there is a Canadian amongst the wounded, the tension builds noticeably. The mood lightens again when we hear that he has only sustained a minor injury to his hand.

No one seems to worry about the two captured and wounded hostile militants. Neither do I. I will do my utmost to provide them with the best possible care when they are on our operating table, but I couldn't care less about what happens to them after that.

The two black dots on the horizon are moving towards us at top speed. It has become a familiar sight. The front helicopter is adorned with a red cross on the nose and the side doors. The other one flies right behind it as security. Today, the second helicopter is also carrying the two bodies of the deceased Afghans. I watch them while I smoke a cigarette. A group of about 30 people are now waiting in front of the hospital's doors for the helicopters to land.

The builders who are constructing a new wing next to the entrance to the hospital have temporarily stopped work. Sitting on the roof under construction they stare at the ever-increasing group of care providers and the approaching helicopters.

They land almost simultaneously. The men and women of the stretcher crew immediately start to move and, crouching down, they walk to the helicopters. The casualties are stretchered out and lifted into the waiting ambulances that will bring them to the hospital.

I put out my cigarette with my foot when the first ambulance stops in front of the hospital's entrance. The doors are opened and the injured Canadian is lifted out of the vehicle. The young man, who has short blonde hair, is lying quietly on the stretcher. While he is carried into the hospital he looks around with sharp, fierce eyes.

On the next two stretchers are the tied-up enemy fighters, and the final two victims lie on stretchers placed on the floor outside the hospital. From the way their heads dangle powerlessly from side to side, we can tell that any help would come too late.

I take a sip of water. I am one of the last ones to enter the hospital. I realise it must be a strange experience for the Canadian to be lying next to the ones who were out for his blood only an hour ago.

The hammering and sawing starts again as soon as I walk through the open door. The guys on the roof have seen enough.

The tip of his left index finger is only connected to the rest by a few fibres. Calmly, the blonde soldier looks at it.

The surgeon tells him he won't be able to save the fingertip.

"I don't think I need to be a doctor to see that, doc!"

The orthopaedic surgeon struggles to keep a straight face when he hears the levelheaded answer.

The Canadian surgery team will remove the top part of his finger, while we will take care of the captured militants in the other operating room.

I look at them and notice how they lie there stoically, not uttering a sound, despite their multiple bullet holes. Their eyes show no emotion whatsoever. The answers they give to the surgeon's questions are translated into short, staccato-like sentences by the fully covered, unidentifiable interpreters.

The detainee who needs medical intervention first is placed on the operating table. During surgery we will explore the trajectory of the bullet and repair the damage it has done. It is still in his body and after localising the bullet, it is surgically removed without any difficulty. The second detainee comes into surgery after a physical checkup in the ER and an imaging examination in the X-ray department. There are two visible wounds on his left leg where bullets entered his body.

What stands out is that there is actually a total of four bullets in his body. Two of these are wedged in his pelvis, but there are no entry wounds. The other two are in his left leg.

"He was probably shot before," the surgeon says after a thorough physical examination. We won't worry about the two bullets that might have been in his body for years. Instead, we concentrate on the two in his leg and we remove the bullets from his body during the procedure.

He wakes up from the anaesthesia as soon as we finish dressing his leg. I stand close to the operating table to prevent him from falling, in case he is unsettled whilst waking up. When he looks at me, a torrent of words comes out of his mouth. I look at the interpreter for help.

"Is he praying or singing?" I ask jokingly.

I am told it is neither of those. When I ask what he is saying, the interpreter says he would rather not translate it verbatim, because it is not appropriate. It chills me to the bone and makes me angry. In a much more heavy-handed way than usual, I slide the patient from the operating table to the stretcher. It appears to hurt him, as another flood of lilting words leave his mouth. I look over at the interpreter again.

"Something about your mother," he volunteers, staring at the ground.

HEAVY LOSSES

"All we could do was stand there and look at it all. Damn, we couldn't do a thing!" With a shaky voice and a trembling bottom lip, I light another cigarette before I start to tell a couple of Dutch soldiers about what just happened. I tell them about today, but also about other events that got to me over the past few weeks. It is quiet at the table when I stop talking. Everyone who has been listening is now staring at the bottom of their coffee cups. "Damn, it has really upset me. I won't ever forget it."

One of the guys crunches up his cup and stares at me for a long time. Then he gets up and strides with big steps to the prefab container. He comes back with a full pot of coffee and pours everyone another cup. He says he can't even imagine what happened and actually doesn't want to either. Some of the others agree with him. I realise that the people here have no idea what is going on only half a mile from here, in the hospital and they won't be the only ones.

It was supposed to be a calm day today. However, it ended up being one of the days that would make me falter years later.

~

When I light the first cigarette early in the morning, I nearly cough up my lungs. I have had a dry, barking cough for a couple of days, due to all the dust. It really takes its toll on your lungs.

This cough is affectionately known as The Kandahar Cough. It is a common phenomenon and something that most of us will suffer from sooner or later. I have caught it too and it would take days before I would be able to smoke a cigarette without turning blue.

I sit myself down at the big picnic table, with in front of me a steaming cup of coffee that is way too strong. I think to myself that, whoever is going to try to get me away from here on my day off, will need to be someone very special. That would happen much sooner than expected.

My beeper sounds halfway through a mind-numbingly boring article in a magazine that is far too old. Multiple casualties are on the way to the hospital. I throw the magazine onto the table and quickly make my way to the hospital.

The Canadian team is finishing a surgery when I walk into the hospital. A child of not even ten years old is on their operating table. The surgical wound, that runs from the sternum down to the pubic bone, is being closed up. It has been a lengthy surgery.

This child was shot and suffers from multiple gunshot wounds. What gets to me is that I am no longer surprised to see an innocent kid in the OR. Even the youngest children are victims of the prevalent war violence. Has the desensitising started now that I don't find this situation strange anymore?

The boy is called Aziz and he would stay in the hospital for a long time, becoming one of the staff's favourite patients.

~

The hairs on the back of my neck stand up when I look at the whiteboard and an icy chill goes through my body when I read that

59

again no less than six Canadian casualties are being flown in. Three other Canadians were killed the day before we arrived in Kandahar. It shook the hospital to its core for quite some time. Now another six are on their way, and they require immediate help. All of them have injuries that have the highest priority, and each and every one of them will need urgent medical intervention.

The interpreter, who was on patrol with these Canadians, is also on his way, but unfortunately he already has the dreaded VSA-status. We won't be able to do anything for him.

"This isn't good. No, this isn't good at all," I hear the emergency doctor say.

A cloud of sorrow descends on us. The hospital is under command of the Canadians and now there are six direct colleagues who have been seriously hurt. Everyone in the hospital feels a strong bond with these unfortunate guys. They are our ISAF colleagues and six of our brothers are on their way.

We all feel we have some making up to do. They need to be saved. At the same time there is an almost palpable fear that we might lose one or more lives again. This is amplified by the fact we have already lost the interpreter.

The hour that follows is like something from a slow-motion film. While we are ready and waiting to take care of the wounded, we gradually receive new pieces of information.

The vehicle with the Canadians was struck during Operation Luger by an RCIED, a *remote controlled improvised explosive device*. It is a roadside bomb that was detonated from a distance. It would have been an enormous blow. The explosive created a crater in the ground which was 32 feet in diameter and over 10 feet deep.

It is this explosion that wounded the six Canadians. Their interpreter died there and then. I prepare myself for the fact that these could be the first casualties whose limbs might be completely blown off. Will we now see the true atrocities of war? Even though we have already witnessed more than our fair share of injuries, I am getting increasingly tense.

The status of the wounded is adapted more than once. Two Canadians have now received the VSA-status. After my next cigarette the status is changed once again. It saddens me when I see that only two casualties seem to be surviving the journey to the hospital. The other four and the interpreter have all died.

"If this continues, there won't be any reason for us to be here at all! Waiting is deadly, literally and figuratively!" The doctor paces up and down restlessly whilst he says this out loud. I hear the frustration in his voice.

On the ward, a young nurse is crying. Everyone is down in the dumps and on edge. I am too. Instead of waiting, I want to do something. Anxiously, I see how the hospital's commander makes his way from the communications centre to write an update on the board.

~

I sniff and bite my lip. I close my eyes tightly to prevent a tear from finding its way down. It is surreal. The commander looks a couple of years older as he walks over to the board and slowly erases all notes.

I just stand here powerlessly and watch how we have just lost six colleagues and an interpreter without being able to do a thing. This is horrible.

When I look up, I see people hugging each other in comfort. Some Canadian colleagues are crying openly and I am deeply touched. I enter the OR and start to clean up all supplies we got ready in preparation, as I quickly wipe away a tear. I don't want people to see that I am emotional.

The hospital's Commander thanks us all for our commitment. This remark doesn't sit well with me. We didn't do anything, damn it, we lost before we even started.

"This will be a *ramp ceremony*, Erik. I'm going, what about you?" people ask.

No less than six coffins, all covered with the Canadian flag, will be carried through a guard of honour made up of soldiers from many different countries. Paying our last respects to the fallen is the least we can do. Carried on shoulders, they will enter the plane that will take them home one last time.

I hope I can be there, that we are not busy performing surgery on people who are more fortunate than those today. As soon as I walk out of the hospital, I go to the phone area in the Dutch camp. I desperately want to ring home and talk about what has just happened.

~

"I went to see the GP today," is the first thing I hear when I get my wife on the phone. "I felt like I couldn't breathe and had a tight chest," she continues.

I am frightened when she tells me this.

Then she tells me that it is probably because of her asthma and that I shouldn't worry. I promise her not to.

Where I had solemnly sworn to myself only a couple of seconds ago that I was going to tell her all the details of my horrendous day, I decide there and then not to mention it now I have heard her news. I actually do the exact opposite and the phone call once again ends up being a short conversation about the usual trivial bits of news. I also ask her how the kids are doing and I am glad that they are doing just fine. After saying goodbye, I hear her disconnect the call and listen to the dial tone.

"When I get home, I will tell her and everyone else about today. Not now, but later, at home. Maybe, but then again, maybe not," I say out loud as I slam the phone down.

The oppressing feeling of losing a match without even kicking a ball stays with me and I just can't let it go.

There are fences covered in black plastic sheets close to the hospital. Behind those is the camp's mortuary. As soon as I see the fences, I wonder how the men and women who work there deal with today's events. I am happy I am not in their shoes. In my head I picture the six heavily mutilated bodies of our fallen brothers. The power of the explosion might have injured them beyond recognition. I try and block out that image. I am not able to do that though and it makes me intensely sad.

I walk past the hospital and the mortuary to the break room. With a cigarette in one hand and yet another bottle of water in the other, I sit deep in thought only to jump up when a surly American soldier unknown to me stomps past. He enters the tent and returns with a can of soft drink. Then he grabs a chair, comes and sits next to me and takes a big sip, followed by a huge burp.

"What a fucking day, in this fucking country, in this fucking climate," he growls. I am not sure if he wants me to respond or not. He doesn't seem to care.

"Not good, man. You don't want to know...," he continues, as if he has just read my mind. It is one of the guys from the mortuary. He explains how he has only a few more weeks to go and that he can't wait until he is back home with his wife and kids.

"I recognise that feeling, but it feels as if I've only been here a short while," I answer.

He looks at me as he takes another sip of his drink and scrutinises me.

"Surgery?" he asks, as I nod in agreement. He groans unintelligibly, then starts to tell me at length about how he has been at this base for over thirteen months. He has seen and experienced it all. Days and even weeks of hardly doing a thing and days like today.

"Everyone in the mortuary would rather not do anything, believe me, but damn, it doesn't often work that way," he says as he scrunches up his empty can.

I see the same empty look in his eyes as I saw in the chaplain's eyes earlier. For a short moment I get the feeling that, at the end of my deployment, I might sit in front of this tent the same way as he is now. Completely desensitised, with a confused expression on my face and a backpack full of experiences.

It is a given that lots of people change during their deployment. I tell myself I can't let that happen. After all, I actually don't do anything different from the work I do back at home. We just don't perform planned surgery here. Instead, we wait hour by hour to find out what the day will bring and one day is better than the other. Today is proof of that.

We sit silently and do nothing but smoke and look at the chaos all around us on this busy military airfield. We see transport planes come and go. I listen to the roar of two fighters taking off. Heavy bombs hang under their wings and they are going hunting. Every once in a while, I hear the annoying zooming of a Predator-drone taking off or taxiing. The war is getting closer and closer.

I didn't sleep well. I don't feel fit, like I have been run over by a train and I keep thinking about yesterday. For those couple of hours everyone at the hospital was breathing the same breath. Although I don't have Canadian blood, I still feel I lost some brothers yesterday. I just can't let it go. Annoyed, I walk over to the hospital and on arrival I immediately feel that what happened yesterday has left a scar. The atmosphere in the hospital is sombre and people seem to be talking more quietly.

The ramp ceremony for the fallen will take place the next day. All who want to be there are welcome to attend, providing we keep our distance. This is so we can be called upon if we are needed to help prevent another one of these ceremonies.

A few hours ago, we received yet another message about a huge attack close by. Immediately we prepare the operating theatres to be able to promptly treat those with the highest priority. The hospital is buzzing with activity. A sombre thought enters my head for a brief moment: I hope these aren't ISAF colleagues again. I quickly suppress that thought.

Around midday a man in police uniform intruded the police headquarters in nearby Spin Boldak. He entered a room where, at that time, nearly all police officers were present. Twenty-two people were, unsuspectingly, enjoying their lunch break. Because of his uniform, he was able to make his way there without being hindered. Once inside, he blew himself up.

The information about the number of casualties changes constantly. Eventually, we hear that there are thirteen fatalities, amongst them the perpetrator. Seven men are injured and three others haven't been found yet. The casualties will be flown to the hospital. I realise there is a chance we will be waiting in vain once again.

I sit with my back against the wall of a bunker behind the hospital. We have just finished organising the final instruments and supplies in the operating room and are ready to go as soon as we are offered any patients. Seven victims are on their way.

In the shades of the bunker, protecting me from the blazing heat, I try to imagine what happened in those last moments in that room which makes me sad and fearful. How would it feel to sit down to eat when a complete stranger suddenly storms into the room to blow himself up? Could that happen here as well? Are we truly safe?

The thudding of the helicopter blades is getting closer.

"Jesus Christ, what is that?" I ask genuinely surprised when I see one of the newly arrived casualties come past. It is an introduction to blast wounds.

The victims who have just come in were all in the room when the suicide bomber transformed himself into a human explosive. The flying debris and the pressure released in the explosion has caused awful blast wounds.

Blood streams from multiple wounds on the first patient's left arm and from his side too. The puddle of blood on the floor under the stretcher is getting bigger and bigger. The nurse who is trying to stop the bleeding nearly slips over and curses out loud.

The holes blown into the patient's body are horrible. The skin and the underlying structures have been completely smashed away and destroyed. The muscular tissue, tendons and nerves are all clearly visible. It is already clear that this patient will need multiple surgeries and we will definitely see him on our table more than once. The others have similar injuries. It has a profound impact on me, not in the least because they all seem to be lying so distressingly still. I expected them to be screaming because of the pain, but each and every one of them is staring at the ceiling. One of the patients pulls a face and utters a stream of unintelligible words when one of the staff lifts his arm which is broken in multiple places. It sounds like the singing from a couple of days ago.

"You are hurting the patient a little bit,' the smiling interpreter translates.

Another patient seems unhurt, suffering from a so-called inhalation trauma. His airways have been burned and a breathing tube gets shoved down his throat as soon as he arrives. After that he is taken straight to Intensive Care Unit. By now, three out of four ICU beds are occupied. I will never forget his face, which is grey and charred with soot, dust and dried blood and with sand and debris in his hair and his beard.

You cannot always see the severity of injuries by looking at the outside. Huge wounds can be impressive, but internal trauma can be a much bigger threat to the patient.

The other victims have all sorts of injuries; different fractures and trauma caused by the flying debris.

We work for a long time. Both our team and the Canadian team are taking care of one after the other wounded policeman. It is already dusk by the time we have our final patient on the operating table. This one has huge gaping wounds on both his arms and legs. Several surgeons are simultaneously performing surgery on multiple parts of his body.

The wounds are rinsed and - where possible - damaged muscles and tendons are repaired. The biggest defect is on his upper arm, showing a gaping hole of about four by six inches and several inches deep.

We have been working on him for quite some time when the surgeon suddenly looks up from behind his mask and asks me for long tweezers. He mutters something I don't understand and continues to work more fanatically than before. He then asks me to hold out some clean gauze in my hand whilst he carefully pulls something out of the wound. Everybody looks on with disbelief when the item appears.

"I believe we have just found our perpetrator. Well, at least a part of him," the surgeon says.

There is a piece of tissue wedged between the tweezers. "It looks like scalp," he continues. He looks at this tissue for a bit longer and then digs a little deeper in the policeman's arm to remove a few more pieces of the suicide bomber.

I have experienced quite a lot, but this is by far the most bizarre thing I have ever seen up to now. I could never have expected that we would be picking pieces of a human out of another human. It goes against everything I consider to be normal.

~

Once all patients have been seen, I go and sit in the bunker behind the hospital again. I am exhausted, physically and mentally. I drink something and gather my thoughts. We are ordered to stay put as there is lots of talk in the hospital about another gunfight between a small unit of the Afghan National Army (ANA) and insurgents, that happened not far from here. After waiting for over an hour for more news about this battle, we find out we don't have to wait any longer, as the gunfight is over. Seven people are injured on the Afghan army's side. These couldn't be evacuated from the scene and that means the case is closed for us.

I have no idea what happens to them. I don't need to know anyway, so I don't ask any questions. All I want to do is rest.

I walk over to my camp. I would love to do nothing more than get in my bed and close my eyes. My plan doesn't work though, because a couple of soldiers stop me for a chat and ask if I want to join them for a cup of coffee or a bottle of water, which I do. We sit at the big picnic table, drink coffee together, have a laugh and within minutes I get bombarded with questions. They are keen to find out how we spend our days in the hospital. They wonder if we are busy, as they have been seeing less and less of us.

I stare at the dregs of the cold coffee in my plastic cup. I swirl it around slowly, like it is a good glass of wine, then I sigh and start telling them about the last couple of days.

"It's not easy as the workdays are getting longer by the day. Other than a constant, daily stream of new patients, all with injuries that are both interesting and horrific, we also perform surgery more than once on many admitted patients."

As I have noticed before, these colleagues don't have a clue either about what is going on in the hospital and I can't blame them for that. As best as I can I explain to everyone who wants to listen that there is actually an insidious war going on right around the corner and that we see the results of this every single day.

I tell them that we experience a lot of misery, without going into too many details. I explain that we have saved many wounded but that we have also lost some patients and how we sometimes lose them without being able to do anything for them at all. I also talk about how we take care of wounded detainees and that we have even removed pieces of a suicide bomber from an injured man's body. People are listening intently and I catch a sombre face here and there.

When I get up to go to bed after I have finished my story, my audience stays put without uttering a word.

I don't sleep a wink, even though I am dog tired.

AREA FIFTY-POO

Our surgical team is moving today. We will say our goodbyes to our trusted tent in the heart of the Dutch encampment, and will be stationed amongst Canadians and Americans.

Yesterday our Canadian colleagues were with us for the last time. The team that relieves them has been working alongside of us for some days now. Even though we have only known our colleagues for a short time, it feels like we have been working together for years. The intensity of all procedures and injuries has helped to blur differences between us meaning we have become close very quickly.

I am in my sweaty scrubs when my Canadian colleague comes to see me. He lights a cigarette and inhales deeply. He is the only smoker in his team. Many times, I have stood with him in exactly this place, behind the hospital, sometimes laughing and joking, other times we would be quiet, lost in thought, mulling over what had just happened.

Without saying a word he places a cold piece of metal in my hand. It is the coin he received from the hospital's commander. It lies heavily in my hand, a token of brotherhood and mutual respect. We have stood shoulder to shoulder to save patients in primitive circumstances. His gesture moves me. Then he firmly pounces me on my shoulder and grins from ear to ear. "Take care, mate! Thanks for the good times. Gotta run, going home, yeehah!"

The encampment we will be housed in is a lot further away from the hospital, but at the same time a lot closer to the *Poo Pond,* the *Shitpit* or *Area Fifty-Poo,* as some colleagues say.

During one of my first morning walks, when it is still relatively cool, I unsuspectingly walk across the airfield. I have just had a long shower and a hearty breakfast after an unsettled night. I feel quite fit this morning and take a really deep breath, which I immediately regret. Because of this one breath the whole world seems to exist of nothing more than the nauseating, fetid smell of a massive, open sewer. It is like a slap in the face and stops me in my tracks. Immediately, my stomach protests and there is a sour taste in my mouth and I have to do my utmost to not spill my breakfast all over my shoes. It is little short of a miracle that I manage to keep it all in. I quickly walk away whilst breathing through my mouth. It seems a distant memory that only half an hour ago I had a shower and smelled fresh. I soon find the cause of this stench, it can't be missed.

To the southwest of the airfield there is a big pool of about 100 feet that serves as an open sewer. All faeces of the, by now more than 20,000, inhabitants of the military base ends up here. It is a big lake of brownish sludge and is fenced off with nothing more than barrier tape and a few warning signs. In various spots on the lake you can see little fountains splashing and bubbling away.

Biohazard. No trespassing. No swimming. I smirk when I read the warning signs. As if I would ever decide to go for a nice swim here.

The smell that spreads over camp is indescribable. The Poo Pond isn't hidden away in some remote corner of the airfield, but actually holds a prominent spot on camp. You never get used to the odour. Ever.

Legend has it that a projectile actually landed in this Poo Pond during one of the many missile attacks on the base. It never exploded, but slowly sank to the bottom of the pond never to be seen again. People have also been placing bets on others swimming across the lake, and some claim that people have actually done that.

Later that day I receive the key to my new sleeping quarters. I get a room in a barracks together with two Canadians who also work in the hospital. The accommodation is quite comfortable, with a functioning internet connection and a television.

I introduce myself to my roommates, a physiotherapist and a staff member of the TOC, the *Tactical Operations Centre*, and we rearrange the room. We talk about the upcoming ramp ceremony. They too will line up during the ceremony for the six fallen soldiers later today.

After I have arranged my side of the room and made it my own, I go for a short stroll around the barracks. I want to try and relax for a little while, but the closer it gets, the more uncomfortable I feel about the upcoming ceremony.

Despite the fact that I won't be lining up with the troops because of the risk of a call out, I strongly feel that I have to be there to pay my respects. It is the least I can do.

My barracks are part of a block of six. When outside, I suddenly hear a faint gurgling and see where it comes from. It is an unfortunate twist of fate that I could have anticipated. The gurgling comes from one of the little fountains that continuously spits out lumpy slop. Our sleeping quarter is only 300 feet away from the Poo Pond.

"Shit!"

FAREWELL TO SIX HEROES

The sun has set.

The transport plane is on the platform with its cargo door open at the back. Hundreds of soldiers of many different nationalities form a guard of honour spanning row upon row in line with the plane. The silence is almost tangible.

I am not lined up with the troops, but am somewhere at the back. My colleague Linda is here too, but I can't see her. I observe everything in silence and hope that my beeper won't go off in the coming minutes.

The six coffins with the remains of the fallen are draped with the Canadian flag. The men who carry them all look tense and sombre, some of them are crying. Many of the soldiers that are lined up are crying too. Even though the fallen soldiers were strangers to most people here, every one of us feels a strong connection with them.

Last in line and right behind the final coffin is a soldier with bagpipes, playing Amazing Grace. The bagpipes' languid tones in its minor key sound across the platform and the sad sound of the instrument chills us to the bone. I am deeply moved by this impressive and respectful tribute.

My eyes are filled with tears when I walk off after the ceremony. I have never experienced anything like this in my life. Ever since that day, I have not been able to listen to the sound of bagpipes without hairs on the back of my neck standing up or shivers running down my spine.

I return to the hospital and grab a chair that I put next to the taxiway in front of the hospital. Feeling sad, I sit down and smoke one cigarette after another.

A huge C-17 Globemaster III transport plane taxis past me. I would pay a lot of money to get on board right now and leave this place.

When the aircraft is on the runway and the sound of the engines swells to a deafening roar, a flare is fired into the air from one of the watchtowers on the edge of the camp. The plane starts to move almost immediately and it takes off steeply, disappearing into the night like a big, black shadow. More flares are fired into the sky from multiple watchtowers and a yellow glow lights up the whole base.

It suddenly hits me and I am scared. I can't shake the thought that our base is being attacked by insurgents. I remember the victims from the suicide bomber's attack on the police station and draw a parallel to the here and now.

In my head I picture a group of insurgents entering the airbase through the gate. They are all dressed in uniforms of the different coalition troops and have been instructed to blow themselves up in the areas packed with coalition forces.

I only manage to relax when the flares are extinguished and I reassure myself there are no sounds of a gunfight or explosions of suicide bombers blowing themselves up.

My hand is on my weapon and as I notice that, I get angry with myself. Annoyed, I push the feeling of fear away and a new feeling emerges: shame. I get up and give the chair an almighty kick. Without looking back, I make my way to my new sleeping quarters.

I am in bed but cannot sleep, because I am annoyed about absolutely everyone and everything. The air conditioning doesn't work properly and there is too much light coming from under the door. My bed is saggy, I have no pillow and the worst of it is that my roommates make too much noise in their sleep. I am feeling restless, so I switch on my flashlight, grab my diary and a pen and start to write. Wearily I scribble down a few notes. I write down the names of the six Canadians who we said goodbye to with such reverence today. Feeling down, I put away my diary so I can try and sleep. I don't sleep at all. I will never forget these heroes, nor this day.

More than seven years later, in 2014, I would suddenly relive this emotional ceremony at full force, resulting in me losing control over myself.

A CONTAINER FULL OF
BODY PARTS

Over the last couple of days rumours have been flying around camp about a big military operation due to start in the Kandahar and Helmand provinces. People talk about it as if a lot is going to happen.

All we can do is hope that it won't have too much of an impact on our hospital, but I realise that might well be wishful thinking. The last weeks have been busy. We don't have a lot more intake capacity and more newly injured are on their way to us today.

Two unfortunate Afghan soldiers are stabilised as soon as they arrive. The first patient has been shot in his stomach and the other one has a tightened tourniquet around his right arm. The bleeding from the huge hole has been stopped.

"Look at that arm, Erik, just look at it," I hear Linda say. Even though she is right next to me, she sounds far away. I can't take my eyes off the patient's arm. Just below the tourniquet is a large, gaping wound. It looks like a large fragment went through the arm and destroyed everything in it on its way. It is a miracle in itself that the arm is still connected to the rest of the body.

One of the surgeons joins us to discuss what we are going to do. He glances over his glasses and confirms our suspicion. "There's no honour in this one, it's coming off."

~

The arm is cleaned before the operation. Linda lifts the affected limb in such a way that I can disinfect it from all angles. It is now clear how badly damaged the arm actually is. There doesn't seem to be any firmness below the elbow whatsoever. It is as if the inside is made of pudding and the arm flops like a rag doll in her hands. Everywhere around me I can hear the clicking of cameras again.

As soon as the arm and the patient have been covered with sterile drapes the surgeons begin the amputation. I assist during the procedure. We work efficiently towards the inevitable moment of the arm being separated from the body.

I am handed the removed limb by one of the surgeons and am surprised by the weight of it. I have assisted numerous times with amputations at home, but it continues to be extraordinary to hold an entire limb and to then dispose of it. I ask Linda to get ready with a double red bag and slowly lower the arm into it. She also seems surprised when she feels the dead weight of it. Then she ties up the bag and places it in the corner of the operating room.

Less than an hour after we started the procedure and after a short search in the logistical labyrinth for the required stump bandage, that somebody relocated once again since the last time we searched for it, the patient is taken to the ward. He weighs several pounds less than before.

~

It is getting busier all the time, not only in hospital but also in my head. Day in, day out we look after patients who are experiencing their worst day ever. I see bodies that have been blown to pieces and lives that are significantly changed in a split second.

Things are getting under my skin and some of those have started to itch. I have only been here for a couple of weeks and I refuse to admit that things have started to get to me.

The image of an Afghan soldier with two severely injured legs from a roadside bomb attack pops into my head. I imagine what it would be like.

As soon as he opens his eyes and looks up, all he sees is strangers, who are wearing surgical caps and facemasks and are bent over him. Bright, blue eyes are staring down at him and he notices their worried looks. Everyone is shouting at each other in a language that is incomprehensible to him. He is overwhelmed by panic and starts to move around frantically, but his body doesn't want to cooperate. Then he looks down and it hits him with full force. Where there used to be two healthy legs, everything below his knees has now been changed into a bloody mass of tissue. Anxiously he looks around. He speaks continually but no one seems to hear him. Then his eyes find a pair of dark eyes and he hears a calm voice he can understand. He starts to talk wildly and it sounds like begging.

"He asks if you can save his legs," the interpreter says. "Without his legs he can't take care of his family. If you can't save his legs, he would rather be dead."

The surgeon listens to the interpreter and takes a quick look at the patient's lower legs.

"Even though we are very good, we have our limitations... Nope, can't save them, not a chance in hell."

I somehow do understand these patients who, as soon as they come in, start to plead with us to do whatever it takes to save their legs. And if we can't do that, could we then please kill them.

In a country like Afghanistan, where a majority of the population is deprived of the most basic facilities like sanitation, it is all about survival of the fittest. Patients whose leg or legs we have to amputate immediately fall outside this category. He won't be able to work for his family any longer, and might have to beg for the rest of his life to survive. He will have to be looked after by his family and will be a burden to them because of it. I doubt if I am helping to do something good here. Is what we offer actual help? Don't we take his future away by saving a patient like him? It seems to me that we save a life, but destroy it at the same time. More than once we go against the clearly expressed wish of the patient. Instead of complying with it, we do all we can to save the life of the injured man. That is what we should do, as we have taken an oath to do whatever we can to save lives, that is what we are here for. But the paradox between saving lives and destroying them simultaneously is in my head now. I don't want to think about it too long, because if I do that, I will doubt what we are doing here even more.

Every surgery we perform produces a huge pile of medical waste. Used surgical gowns and gloves, bloodstained surgical drapes, gauze dressings and packaging material of all used instruments. At the end of the procedure everything is crammed into big bags and deemed to be potentially contaminated waste. It needs to be stored separately and burnt at a later date.

Another procedure applies to amputated limbs though. They have to be taken in red bags to a white, refrigerated container just outside the hospital, where they will be stored until the patient is discharged from the hospital.

I put the key in the padlock of the cooled container's big and heavy door and it opens with a click. There are three waste bags on the floor right in front of me, containing waste from the last procedure. The container's door is hard to open and squeaks. I pull it open just enough to squeeze myself and the bags through it.

Before I step into the container I fill my lungs with air and hold my breath until I step out again. Only then I breathe in again and can immediately taste and smell the disgusting Poo Pond odour, that is absolutely everywhere on camp. But I prefer that smell over the one in the container.

The bags with medical waste are piled high in this storage. There is a cooling system, but it isn't equipped to deal with the temperatures here and that is why there is always a pungent smell of old blood and decomposition. To the right there is a stack of double red bags, all labelled and containing amputated limbs. There were only a few of those the first time I stepped into the container, but now there is quite a pile and only once in a while a few disappear. When an Afghan patient is discharged, the bag with the correct label is found in the pile of limbs and handed over to the patient or his family to take home.

Later during my deployment, when the mountain of bags had grown enormously, it became more and more of a morbid task to search bag after bag in that reeking, dark container for the one labelled with the correct patient number. Even though I know they are, to this day I sincerely hope that those labels were actually all correct and that every patient received the right limb upon discharge.

It never feels good to go there late at night to dispose of the waste. I would open the door and throw the normal waste as far into the back of the container as possible, preferably whilst still standing outside, as inside death was all around. I would place the waste from patients right around the corner, so that I don't have to go further into the container. Then I would hurry outside, retching whilst walking back to the light of the hospital.

Having closed the door and locked the padlock, I wander back to the OR. It has been another long day, with multiple casualties, who we have helped in one way or another. Injuries caused by violence seem to become the norm and I don't seem to be surprised anymore when we see people with gaping wounds or others who have been partially blown up.

I meet the chaplain in passing. He smiles at me and asks me how it is going. I think about it for a moment and tell him I am getting used to the gruesomeness of war, but not to losing a game once in a while. No, not to that, never to that.

"I hate losing, padre."

"The one thing that is really important is that you don't lose yourself on the way," he says when I walk off. That surprises me. It is confirmation for me that people can come back differently from a mission. I always told myself that if I would change because of my deployment, it would only be because of the wealth of experience I had gained and I would return an enriched man.

I know the stories of people who go crazy. Some straight away, others not until years later, but that only happens to others, right? I won't let that happen to me, because the work I do is basically the same as I do at home, only the circumstances are different.

Questions pop into my head. Am I also piling on the pressure? Am I under a lot of stress? If I am honest to myself I have to answer yes to those questions.

I was scared the night the flares were shot up into the sky, when I thought the base was under attack. I was sad and defeated on the day those six Canadians and their interpreter couldn't be saved and I have felt so cynical when seeing heavily injured patients. It is awful what people can do to each other.

I will have to see what is going to happen next. For me, it is more and more about surviving. Day to day. Every 24 hours, the kids at home eat one sweet each from the jar that is getting emptier every day as another day gets crossed off on the calendar. I can't wait to go back to my wife and children. I miss them like hell..

WOUNDED COLLEAGUES

I feel I am slowly falling ill. The last couple of days I have been coughing my lungs out and have had flulike symptoms. Physically I soon feel better, but I can't seem to empty my head that easily anymore.

Despite the fact that the most horrendous injuries are now becoming the norm, a few events stay with me. I deliberately choose not to discuss this with the people in my team, because I don't want them to think that I am weak. In their eyes I am the tall, jolly, and sometimes downright oafish joker who wanders around the hospital in his big, yellow clogs. It is a role that suits me down to the ground and I play it with gusto. However, it is just a role I play as I prefer to keep what really goes on in my head to myself. I don't discuss my deeper feelings, my worries and my fears with anyone, not even with Linda.

On top of all the misery we see, the threat from the outside is increasing too. Stories are doing the rounds about hostile militants who have been able to get their hands on a batch of uniforms from the Afghan army and police. Dressed in those uniforms, they are planning attacks on police stations, army bases, market squares and off course ISAF-locations. That is food for thought.

Everyone in a Dutch uniform with an ISAF patch is dealt a heavy blow, as no less than eight soldiers have been wounded in a suicide bombing at the bazaar in Deh Rawod. One of them is in critical condition, the other seven are stable. A total of thirteen inhabitants of the village were killed in the attack and another 30 or so people were injured.

We are due to receive more information about our wounded colleagues tonight. I smoke some cigarettes as I let the news sink in and I suddenly understand the oppressive feeling that our colleagues in the hospital felt when some of their countrymen were fatally injured.

The critically wounded soldier has already been in surgery in Helmand. Three other casualties have been stabilised and are being cared for in the Dutch Role-2 hospital near Tarin Kowt in Uruzgan and the other four are stable too. They will be transferred to Kandahar tonight from where they will be flown back home.

"Let's agree never to meet each other at my work," I said days before to a few men and women who leave the base daily to go on patrol.

I suddenly realise that the people I spoke to that day were all on their way to Deh Rawod. Out of all people it surely can't be them who have been injured? I really hope that I won't see any familiar faces tonight.

On top of this dramatic news, we also hear that soon a weekly talk will be organised for all Dutch personnel. There will be several officials at this gathering who will give briefings about the current state of affairs, the threat level, any imminent actions and more general information. It is a welcome addition to the existing provision of information. One of the specialists of our team immediately proposes to tell the others about the ins and outs of the hospital at one of those meetings, as not many people know about the work we do. This is so we can show them that we work hard here every day, and that there are many more victims than most people at camp would realise. Apart from that, it would also be a great opportunity to explain that the life and limb saving surgery we perform here is a major thing.

Although my body still aches - my voice is hoarse because of the coughing and on top of that I have an infected eye - I perform my tasks at the hospital and in the OR to the best of my ability while playing my role as joker at the same time.

At the moment, our surgery programme consists of some patients that have been in the hospital for a while. Most of them have blast wounds. Almost 80% of patients who end up on our operating table have this sort of injury and we also see lots of casualties with bullet wounds.

The blast wounds are caused by explosions of landmines, suicide attacks and roadside bombs. An explosion like that doesn't only partially or completely destroy a victim's limbs, it also bombards a body with debris, dust and sand. These wounds have to be cleaned over and over again.

During so-called *debridement,* infected and dead tissue is cut away to create a healthy wound environment, so it can heal. It often seems to be one of the only things we do. Every day we flush large wounds and we work on them surgically, like today. We take care of patients we have already seen in our operating room before. This is, as already explained, an essential difference with what we do at home, where of course it does sometimes happen that due to complications, a patient comes back for a follow-up procedure, but here it appears to be nearly protocol.

When the last patient leaves our OR and the programme looks clear for the next hour, I am able to get out of the hospital for a bit. I sit down at the tent behind the hospital.

I look up when a car stops in front of the veterinary practice, right next to the tent where I extinguish my cigarette and throw away my empty bottle of water. A cage is lifted from the car, and placed on the floor. People start to crowd around it. I am curious too, so I get up and walk over. Behind the bars of the cage we see what looks like a wild dog, a beautiful creature. It looks a bit like our dog I took away shortly before I left for Afghanistan. It looks around wildly with its tail between its legs, trembling with fear and foaming at the mouth.

The tall vet comes from his practice and takes a quick look at the dog. From his breast pocket he whips out a syringe and without saying a word, he empties it into the dog. Then he turns around and walks back to his tent. It takes a while before the dog starts to sway. A few seconds later it collapses. Some soldiers, who were watching too, start to chuckle. They laugh about this animal dying. I understand it had to be put down, as it was ill and posed a danger to the health on the base, but this is not my kind of entertainment. I turn around and walk back to the hospital.

~

"They're on their way," Linda says.

It is early in the evening. We have been performing surgery all afternoon and it takes a moment before I realise she is talking about the injured Dutch colleagues.

One by one the casualties are brought in, I only see them for a moment. It is quite tough to deal with the fact that there are now patients in the hospital we can address in our own language. These are our people, our brothers and sisters. I only stay at the hospital for as long as I have to. There are lots of people attending and I feel I am in the way. There is not much we can do other than wishing them a good flight home.

Slowly but surely, I am starting to feel that we haven't seen the worst of this war yet.

Together with Linda I walk from the hospital to the sleeping quarters and chat about our work. We have worked together in the same hospital at home for more than one and a half years, but we don't really know anything about each other. Before I was transferred to that hospital, I worked in another one for three years where I had a great time at the surgery department. I would go to work with a smile on my face every single day, and I would come back home with a grin from ear to ear. That all changed when I was transferred to the other side of the country.

From the very first day I walked around my new place of work with a face like thunder. Despite brave attempts from a couple of colleagues I wasn't interested in integrating at all. I wanted to do my own thing and didn't want to get involved. When I wasn't in the operating room I would be in the smoking area. So, there wasn't a click with Linda either. In fact, I had never really spoken a word to her. I simply never made the effort to get to know her or my other colleagues.

In Afghanistan, we are stuck with each other, day in, day out. We have a lot of time to talk during the long working days and the free hours. I only notice now that Linda is a great colleague; she is driven and precise, has team spirit and above all she is a lovely person. I courteously admit that I was completely wrong about her.

NEWS FROM HOME

"Take a hand truck when you go to the mail room," Linda chuckles. She is smiling broadly at me with a pile of post cards and a package in her hands.

The post has just arrived, what a wonderful moment. It is obvious there is quite a lot for me and I suddenly understand all the stories from soldiers about how mail is a moment to look forward to. I hurry over and see lots of smiling faces around me.

People walk out of the door with piles of post and packages. There is also quite a mountain in front of me. Packages and cards from home. As if I am at the sales, I grab everything.

I sit down at a big picnic table, and open the packages and envelopes one by one. I am overwhelmed by a warm feeling.

My wife has made foot- and handprints of our boys on big sheets of colourful paper, and they have also made a drawing themselves. I smile from ear to ear. After I have looked at them for a while and have read all cards and letters more than once, I walk to my sleeping quarters where I stick all cards and drawings carefully on my wall. For a moment, but just for a moment, I feel a little closer to home.

The last couple of days have been hectic. We perform surgery on a lot of patients. Their injuries vary from minor to unrecognisably maimed. It happens more often now that we are operating with both teams in both theatres at the same time. This means we aren't able to rest as much as usual and this takes its toll on me.

We have mainly operated wounds on arms, legs, lower abdomens and faces. We notice that only a relatively small number of patients comes in with chest wounds. To a large extent this is thanks to the flak jackets that are being worn. Patients are often brought in covered head to toe in a thick layer of clotted blood, dust and other types of dirt while the torso is completely clean and undamaged. These vests most definitely contribute to the survival chances of the patient. On the other hand, it means that if a patient does survive an attack, sometimes multiple limbs are blown off, or will have to be amputated.

I wonder what would be worse. What would I want? While running earlier this week I passed an area with all sorts of remnants of vehicles. It was obvious that these were hit by landmines, roadside bombs or other explosives. They had been transformed to warped pieces of metal and I wondered then what it would be like to be a soldier in one of those during an explosion. I dread to think what it is like to have to leave the base in one of those armoured coffins. They risk their life for a country that, in my eyes, doesn't want to be helped at all.

It must be a nightmare for victims to notice that they can't move, because their legs don't want to any longer or because they are simply not there anymore. I try and imagine the panic that ensues at the moment of an attack, the screams and the excruciating pain and I also think about what it would be like to wake up in hospital and find out that your arms and legs have been amputated. What would there be left to live for? Would I want to be saved if I had to miss my arms and legs? No, I would curse the people who had saved me for the rest of my pathetic life.

"Kill me if I ever have to give up my arms and legs," I hear so often. To then deny his plea and cooperate with amputating patient's limbs and keeping them alive.

That is exactly what we have done today. Other than a couple of soldiers with minor injuries another young soldier was brought in. The injury to his right arm was so severe that we had to amputate it. Well, at least we saved another life today, I think sarcastically.

≈

"I've had your post today and I am so happy with it," I say cheerfully to my wife on the phone. "Please give the boys a big hug from me."

I don't tell her about how busy we have been lately, with multiple casualties, long days and short nights.

My wife then tells me that she still gets a tightness in her chest at times, and that it doesn't seem to go away yet. She sounds a bit worried.

She is not stupid of course. She does watch the news at home. Would they have mentioned how unsettled this region is or maybe she has heard about the attack that wounded a couple of Dutch soldiers? Perhaps she worries a lot more than she is letting on. If that is the case, we both portray what the other wants to see.

After the phone call I wait for Linda. Together we walk back to our camp. The sun is now high overhead and the wind is getting stronger. I won't be surprised if we will soon get a sand or dust storm.

As soon as we walk around the corner, we are stopped in our tracks by a Dutch flag that is fluttering boldly in the strong wind. It is flying at half-mast. Simultaneously we reach for our beepers. The screens are empty. We haven't missed any notifications.

Some colleagues tell us that a Dutch soldier has died. It is the young man who was severely injured in the suicide bombing in Deh Rawod.

He was flown back home and passed away from his injuries yesterday in the Central Military Hospital. Although I didn't know the guy, I feel sad as he was one of us.

Upon hearing this news I no longer feel like hanging out at the tent in the Dutch camp and walk back to my sleeping quarters. I tell my roommates that we have suffered a fatality. The news hits them too. The connection between ISAF colleagues is tangible.

It is dark in the bedroom. My roommates are sleeping. The air-conditioning blows a constant stream of cold air into the room, making the hairs stand up on the back of my neck and giving me goosebumps. I feel my way to my headlamp, switch it on, grab my green diary and start to write: lieutenant T.K., 24 years old, injured at the bazaar in Deh Rawod in a suicide attack, died 12th July 2007. I pull the blanket a bit higher and sigh. It takes ages before I fall asleep.

THE SHARP EDGE

I long for peace and quiet.

I notice that the last couple of long days really got to me. I am dead tired, I am longing for a good night's sleep. Far too often we have been operating with both teams in both theatres at the same time.

Several days we don't get to bed till really late and more than once it is the middle of the night when we finally stop working. We haven't had enough time to rest. Then there is the added pressure of being on call, which makes me feel like I never have any free time.

I also feel kind of caged in at base, as I am in a fenced and heavily-guarded camp, which we can't leave. There is no freedom of movement and this oppressive feeling would take on a tough new meaning only a day later.

~

We have just been notified of an injured child. It is a boy of about twelve years old who is on his way to hospital and he is suffering from a serious stab wound. That is strange, I think. Why is he coming here, as it doesn't seem to be related to the coalition troops' combat operations. Another question, but just as valid, is how a young child like him can ever be a victim of a stabbing. I am once again amazed at the apparent idiocy in this country.

He was initially taken to the local Mirwais hospital with a stab wound to the forehead. The surgeons there didn't know what to do with him and our hospital was able to take him. He will return to Mirwais for after treatment and further care. I am curious, as it sounds like it is a severe injury and everyone is prepared for the worst-case scenario. It is pure barbarity to so severely hurt an innocent child. What sort of culture has no regard for age at all?

I am taken aback when the boy comes in on a stretcher. He is motionless. A big, bright white bandage is wrapped around his head. Bewildered I realise that, under all of these bandages, the knife must still be in the boy's head. I feel sickened, my legs are weak and it takes effort to actually keep upright. I am speechless.

When the last bandages have been removed, a surreal scene unfolds. A knife protrudes from the boy's forehead. It has been pushed into his forehead at an angle all the way up to the handle. It is overwhelming and I feel a big, dark cloud hanging over me, ready to explode.

What unbelievably stupid people must live in this country to brazenly sort out children with a knife? How can someone consciously consider grabbing a massive knife to then ram it, down to the handle, into the head of a 12-year-old boy? This sort of action is not a threat, it is an action aimed to kill. A stab wound to an arm or a leg is bad enough, but to push a knife into a skull with full force is simply barbaric.

Rage is building, one I can hardly control and I wish I could break something now, preferably the person who did this and with my bare hands.

I suddenly remember a story of my uncle, who spent a big part of his life in South Africa and Namibia. He was the director of a hospital and saw a lot of victims of violence every day. He once told me about a young guy who was brought in with an axe wound. They didn't need to do any additional examinations to come to that diagnosis as it was still stuck in his back. Half an hour later a man entered the hospital and asked, without shame, if they could give him back his axe.

It makes me realise that there are actually places in this world where a human life isn't worth anything at all and today I add Kandahar to this list. I just don't understand it and I hope I will never come to understand it either.

Later on, I speak to one of the interpreters and ask him about the circumstances. He tells me that the boy was present at a fight between two adult men on the streets. The fight threatened to get out of hand and one of them fled. The other man thought the boy, who was watching, was his opponent's son and therefore the next in the bloodline. Without mercy, he punished the child as if he was another adult. With brute force and without compassion he pushed the knife into the boy's head and left him to die. The boy was immediately taken to the local hospital. The doctors there quickly realised they were not equipped to deal with this. Eventually they asked ISAF if our hospital would be able to offer the necessary help to this innocent victim.

"But was this boy actually the son?" a nurse asks the interpreter.

He looks down for a moment after which he answers.

"No."

The boy had all the luck in the world on this warm evening in July. If he had been a cat he would have lost eight of his nine lives that night. He came off relatively lightly. Even though the knife was rammed into his forehead, it hardly hit the brain. It did however go behind the eye and got pushed into the cavity.

This case is damn typical for the entire deployment. Everything I do here seems so pointless. Together with others I am committed to our patients, and to the greater good, which are the country that should eventually become more stable and the life of the inhabitants that should be safer. And now this. If people treat each other like this, surely they don't want to live any different from how they did in the Middle Ages. What am I still doing here? I want to leave as soon as possible, back to civilisation and back to my family and friends, back to the ones I love.

I have to perform this role for another couple of weeks and keep it going till September, and then leave as quickly as I can - to never come back again. Go home and forget that I have ever been here, forget about everything I have seen and done. I want to sit my kids on my lap, tell them that daddy loves them and that I will always do everything I can to protect them.

∾

I am unable to swallow even one mouthful of my dinner. I will have to forget about that today then. I just want to rest and think about nothing at all. I need to be with other countrymen for a while and I want to talk about nice things rather than tell them about what I have just seen. They might have had a good day and I want to hear all about it. Just a light-hearted chat, good company, a cup of coffee, a bottle of water and a cigarette. I don't mention the boy, but discuss other patients we have seen before, telling them about the severity of injuries, but trying not to give too many details. I also tell them that it does sometimes happen that we can't save patients and I notice the listeners are impressed by my story. It is quite a relief to talk about this with neutral people.

At the hospital we hardly discuss the impact of our experiences. Even after major events we don't really evaluate. At home it is the most natural thing in the world to be 'cuddled to death' by colleagues after a particularly tough case. Evaluating events is really important, there are even special teams for that. There is no evaluating here whatsoever. Whether that is policy, or us as a team, or me, I am not sure. It simply doesn't happen.

I drink a couple of bottles of water and as many cups of coffee. They are strong and old as per usual. I quickly ring home, and explain that we did work today, although we weren't on shift, but that I can still manage it all.

"Don't worry about me, love. Work is interesting and I apply lots of sunscreen all the time. Please send my love to everyone and give the boys a massive kiss and cuddle from me."

As soon as I finish the call, I want to kick myself. Once again, I pretend everything is alright while I have just experienced something that has deeply touched me. I curse and stomp off to my sleeping quarters.

Later that day, I stare at the sky as I am sitting on one of the plastic chairs in front of my room. The sun is setting on Kandahar. However dark the place is, it still is beautiful to see that big, red ball sink behind the mountain ridge. Silently I look at it and for a while I don't think about anything else.

~

I am less and less surprised by most injuries. Even the most horrendous injuries that I see on a daily basis almost seem 'normal'. I regularly joke harshly about those injuries and the victims no longer bother me that much. I also seem to feel different levels of empathy for different patients.

I don't seem to struggle with performing surgery on a captured hostile fighter. I simply don't feel a lot of empathy towards them. I feel more when we help Afghan soldiers and policemen, because these men were willing to stand up and contribute to change in this country. Civilians have an even bigger impact on me. These are the so-called innocent victims of war.

Up to now we haven't really had to welcome many wounded civilians to our operating room. The majority of our patients has been Afghan police and military.

The ones that have the biggest impact on me are our brothers and sisters from the coalition forces and also the most vulnerable in this barbaric culture. Especially children, because we can say with near certainty that their injuries were deliberately caused by someone close to them. It is the same with women. The severity of the injuries and the insane reasons for these victims' injuries make it all the more dramatic.

Don't think about it too much, I try and tell myself. Only another couple of weeks and then I will be home again. Just do what needs to be done and then leave, to never look back again.

Today I again wasn't able to find the peace and quiet I have been longing for. I smile briefly when I see my bedroom's wall. It is covered with my kids' drawings and all the cards I have received making the wall look like a patchwork of colourful craft projects. I listen to some music and before I know, I fall into a restless sleep.

The hospital's doors open with a bang. The heat from outside invades the building. In the distance sounds the monotonous thudding of helicopter blades. A cloud of dust spreads when the helicopter takes off and disappears out of sight. Another group of victims has just been dropped off at the hospital. One by one three injured policemen on stretchers are carried inside.

Their groaning and shouting breaks the silence. It was calm at the hospital before those double doors opened. It was the typical calm before the storm. All hospital personnel are ready for whatever the never-ending war in southern Afghanistan throws up. Everyone is here to take care of the injured, who are experiencing their worst day ever.

The screams of the patient are blood-curdling. The police car he was travelling in hit a landmine. The attack happened just a few miles away from our camp. I suddenly realise that the blast we heard earlier this morning almost certainly was the explosion of this mine.

The hospital slowly fills with the now familiar scent that every victim of an explosion seems to be carrying: a sickening mixture of diesel, gunpowder, blood and burnt flesh.

"My legs," the young policeman mutters over and over again, "don't take them off. Please, don't take them off. Without my legs I won't be able to live."

His right leg is severely damaged. It is positioned in an unnatural angle below the knee. His trousers have been torn to pieces and the left leg doesn't look much better. The rest of his body is covered in a grey layer of sand, dust and dried blood. It is obvious that he won't be going out on patrol ever again.

The second patient has similar injuries. Because the explosion took place under the car, both his legs were destroyed in a matter of seconds. At the same time another patient is carried to the hospital. With every step the stretcher crew takes, his head bobs powerlessly from side to side. The stretcher is placed in front of the hospital's door. As soon as it touches the floor, his head drops back and his arms spread out. His eyes are half-open and it is as though he is staring up to the sky, wondering what has happened to him. There is no light in his eyes anymore; he is beyond help.

Although losing lives is part and parcel of the work at the hospital in war-torn Afghanistan, I never get used to it.

The two men who have just been brought in have had more luck. They survived the trip to the hospital and are placed in the emergency room, where doctors and nurses immediately start to identify the injuries and work to stabilise them. After this first assessment they are going into surgery in order of severity and that is where we step in.

The following hours we try to save the lives and legs of both patients. We, as the surgical team, will largely determine the future of these police officers. When the first patient is on the operating table, we can see the damage and all its painful details. The right leg is so heavily damaged that we already know it can't be saved and we really have to pull out all the stops to save his left leg.

During the many hours of surgery that follow, the operating room gradually changes into a battlefield. The blue surgical drapes slowly discolour to a deep red shade. They have reached their maximum absorption capacity, they are saturated and blood drips onto the floor. The puddle under the operating table is steadily growing.

We work for a long time and do everything we can, but we aren't able to save either leg. We amputate them both below the knee.

The second patient goes into surgery straight after him. We manage to save his right leg, but the left leg is so badly injured that it is amputated below the knee.

At the end of the surgery we remove all the drapes from the patient. This is when we notice the human being again. We have just been taken care of very young men in the prime of their lives. Men who devoted themselves to rebuilding the country in their roles of police officers. They were willing to stand out from the crowd and for that they have had to pay a high price.

"Erik," a colleague says, "I came over here to help patients and to make them better. What is this shit?"

I look up and nod.

Before I came to Afghanistan I had the same idealistic views. I didn't really count on surgeries like the ones we just performed. Surgeries through which patients do live, but which don't give me a good feeling. Without remorse we have just amputated their legs and have put them in rubbish bags, like they were dead weight. One well-placed cut of the amputating knife changed these proud police officers into crippled men. Men who are in their twenties. My colleague is right. What is this misery?

I wonder how these guys will react when they wake up. What will they think and feel when they look down? Where their legs used to be are now just stump dressings. I don't actually want to know, as I feel ashamed and guilty.

That bad feeling intensifies when, after tidying the operating room, I walk through the hospital with two full red waste bags. A cute looking nurse smiles at me when I walk past but her look changes as she quickly glances at the bags. She pulls a disgusted face. I quickly look away. I understand her as I would do the same, however right now she makes me feel like I am an executioner.

≈

This should have been my day off, but we were called in to save people. We succeeded, but at the same time we also ruined lives. Again, I haven't managed to relax at all today.

It has been like this for weeks. With a smile and my wooden shoes I walk through the hospital, telling jokes and playing tricks, but inside I have had enough. I am done with seeing the most gruesome injuries day after day. Although I play the clown, I am troubled by what I see and do. I need to try and hang on for another couple of weeks.

Performing surgery on an unwavering stream of heavily wounded and mutilated war victims has started to take its toll. It is getting more and more hectic in the hospital and at the surgery department. I am sometimes personally affected by what I see and experience. I realise that people intentionally harm others and that the universal cliché is true: war brings out the worst in people.

STRUCK A NERVE

'The Week in Review' is going to be organised for the first time tonight in Dutch Corner. Briefings will be given about, amongst other things, the security situation, some current matters and ongoing operations in the region. It is organised to get more insight into what everyone is doing on base. There is also a slot for a presentation about the work we do at the hospital.

A few days ago, someone casually asked if we actually did anything at the hospital. Perhaps he imagined we mainly work on our tan during the day. If only he knew.

For this occasion, one of the specialists has prepared a slideshow about the goings-on at the hospital. This has one goal only, to make everyone present aware of the fact that we perform lots of surgical procedures every day.

We have already watched the short film and some of the images don't leave much to the imagination. Personally, I would have chosen less explicit images. I wonder if the audience is ready to see patients who have lost both lower legs, or detailed pictures of dramatic injuries. If the presentation is meant to be hard-hitting and show people what war surgery is all about, it is guaranteed to be a success.

Before we go to Dutch Corner we still have an afternoon of taking care of heavily injured casualties ahead of us. The first patient has nearly lost his entire bottom jaw. We work for hours to reconstruct it. The second patient has wounds all over his body. These are rinsed, seen to, and once we are done with all the procedures, bandaged up.

The sun has already set on Kandahar. Dutch Corner is a hive of activity. The colourful hut is jam-packed. We make our way through the crowd and when we arrive at the bar I pour myself a cup of coffee. As soon as I take my first sip, I realise it was a mistake to choose coffee. My face obviously shows exactly what I feel, as people around me laugh at the face I pull. Soon enough we are chatting to a group of people and it promises to be a nice get-together.

The briefing starts with a comprehensive presentation about roadside bombs that are found in many places along the main roads in the vicinity and the neighbouring areas. Whether these have been found before they exploded isn't mentioned. There has been a sharp increase in the number of attacks in the city of Kandahar and there doesn't seem to be an end to them either.

The news that hostile militants have been able to get their hands on a batch of uniforms of the Afghan forces is being confirmed. Their plan is to wear them to get close to their targets. They would be able to spread death and destruction relatively easily with the help of those uniforms.

Finally, it is confirmed that a large operation will start in the provinces of Helmand and Kandahar in the near future. There has been a lot of rotation at the base lately. More troops than ever seem to populate the camp. The focus of the operation will be on Helmand. This could potentially put extra pressure on the medical facilities of both our hospital and the English Role 3 hospital in Helmand. You have got to crack a few eggs to make an omelette. The information session goes on for longer than planned, so it is decided that our specialist's film is postponed till the next meeting.

After the briefing I sit with Linda and some others at the big picnic table. We drink coffee and water and talk a bit about the briefing. We all agree that it was a valuable addition to the information supply and it is also a good opportunity to speak to other people than just our direct colleagues.

A soft whooshing sound suddenly cuts through the quiet night. The hairs on my arms and in my neck suddenly stand on end. I recognise it from my early days in my military service. Years ago, I was stationed as a medic at an army base, also known as the A.S.R., *Artillery Shooting Range*. The firing range is in one of the most beautiful parts of the Netherlands. Large artillery would be firing grenades across the A.S.R. daily. They flew over the camp to land several miles away in the target area. There would be a short silence after every shot. After that the faint whooshing sound of the grenade flying overhead could be heard, followed by another short silence and the rumble of the impact in the distance. The memory of it is anchored in my mind.

This evening I hear that whooshing sound again. As soon as I feel the trembling in my body, all my senses sharpen. I chuck away my plastic cup and my instinct takes over. I throw myself on the floor onto my stomach in the sharp gravel. "Take cover! Get down!"

A short silence is followed by a huge blast. The ground is shaking. It definitely is a direct hit on the base and very close. Immediately after the blast there is another whooshing sound and another impact, followed by yet another. Then there is silence. I get back up and look around me to see others doing the same. We start running to the nearest bunker. During that sprint I hear and feel two more impacts. Every blast makes me cringe. Tripping over my own feet I reach the bunker.

By now it is filled with a big group of other people. They are all talking and some are laughing out loud. I stagger and look for some support from the bunker's wall. Sweat is running down my face.

Why isn't the siren going? With shaking hands I try to roll a cigarette. Another soldier has just lit one and notices me struggling with my roll-up. He smiles at me and offers me a filter cigarette which I gratefully accept.

I light it, inhale deeply, and exhale even deeper. I am terrified and at the same time an unstoppable anger is growing within me. I realise that I am wearing a uniform with an ISAF patch, which makes me a legitimate target in the eyes of the enemy. There has just been an attempt to attack the base. It feels as if they have tried to bomb me personally though.

Damn, I have been sent to this country full of morons to help and save lives and I am here to do good things. As a way of thanking me for this they now try and kill me. Will there be more grenades? When will it be safe again? And why are some people still walking around? As of now this war is personal.

"Assholes!"

Halfway through my cigarette the air raid sounds. It goes straight through me. We would regularly hear this piercing sound and the tinny voice resonate through the speakers. The sound of it or of a projectile flying above gives me the chills every single time. It scares me.

The first couple of times the alarm sounds I am almost certain that this incoming projectile has my name written all over it and I am scared of dying. Scared that I won't see my wife and children again. Or even worse, that they have to keep going without a daddy and a husband. Damn, I just want to go home.

When the *all clear* is given, I wander back to Dutch Corner. I go back to the place where moments ago I dived under the table to lie flat on my stomach.

I talk about what just happened with Linda and some others. It has scared them too. A normal reaction to an abnormal situation. It has actually more than frightened me, but I am keeping up appearances. I am not showing it, but I feel that my hands are still shaking. If I try to have another roll-up, the cigarette paper rips. I swear loudly and this makes me even angrier than needed. I get up from the bench and hurry inside, grab a bottle of water and breathe deeply. I man up, because I don't want the others to notice.

After rejoining them at the picnic table for a while, I walk back to my room and I talk about the missile attack with my roommates. As they have already been at Kandahar Airfield for months they are used to it and seem unaffected. The cogs in my head however are turning at full speed when I am in bed a bit later.

Kandahar Airfield has the same surface area as a small town. There are about as many inhabitants as in my hometown, so statistically, the chance that one of those missiles lands on me is negligible. But somehow it still feels as if they are aimed at me in particular. The relative feeling of security has been completely wiped away with just a few heavy hits from these incoming projectiles. I feel unsafe and I am fed up. They can all get screwed here.

All the wrong clichés I heard from others have suddenly become real for me. I jokingly said it myself before my deployment: "Withdraw from there and supply weapons to each and everyone who wants to buy them. Then we'll at least make some money from it. Build a wall around it! Bomb it, make it into a sandpit!"

They don't want to be helped. And that is quite convenient, because I don't want to help them anymore.

This day has hit me like a bomb. I crawl into bed, but not before I ring my family. It is my father-in-law's birthday and I congratulate him and quickly speak to my wife and kids who are visiting him. I hope they won't hear the trembling in my voice, as I tell them we have

104

been nice and busy today, but that I am very tired and that I will go to bed now.

I lie awake for a long time, staring at the ceiling and listening to every little sound that could well signal imminent danger. My senses are in full battle mode. After a little while one of my roommates starts to snore uncontrollably and for the first time ever, the sound seems to be strangely comforting. I still can't sleep though.

PROTECTED OR TRAPPED

More than once, I have felt like I am trapped. The camp is really big and heavily guarded which should give me a feeling of safety, even though it is right in the heart of Taliban territory. It doesn't.

During my daily run I am reminded of the fact that dangers are around the corner. When I jog onto the runway and look left I see barbed wire. There are red, triangular signs attached to it in several places. A picture of a skull, Arabic writing with under it the warning: mines.

The fence is only fifteen feet away from the path I am running on. It is an ominous feeling, but also makes me feel protected at the same time. If there are still landmines, people from outside can't just enter the camp. They would announce themselves in advance with a big bang, I think sarcastically.

On the first day, this feeling of relative safety was already affected though, when we were welcomed to 'the base that gets shot at most in the whole of Afghanistan'. Kandahar Airfield definitely earned that title last night. I no longer feel protected, but trapped like a rat.

There is no freedom to do what we like, but hostile fighters can freely fire their missiles from the mountain ridge over to the airport. I am trapped, a sitting duck, and it frightens me to death. It is slowly making me ill.

THE BUTTON IS PUSHED

When I wake up I feel different from the days before. The fear of a new missile attack stays in my system. I no longer sleep solidly and don't feel rested when I wake up.

Before my deployment I told myself and everyone dear to me, that I would be in a safe place. I realise that isn't true. Even Kandahar Airfield with all its facilities isn't a safe place. Although I don't have to go out and look for danger, like the men and women who step out of the base daily, there is definitely a danger. And that feeling of threat has nestled itself deep within me.

I am angry at myself for being so scared and furious with myself because I am frightened to death whilst others don't even seem to care. They are probably the ones who have been here so long that being shot at has become normal. They already know that the chance they will get hit is negligible. In the meantime, I am not even able to roll myself a reasonable cigarette because my hands shake so much. But I also experience a boundless rage aimed at everyone 'in a dress' who fires missiles at us.

I am here in this godforsaken country, in the scorching heat, and I do everything I can for the wounded. I help in saving lives and limbs. It doesn't matter what patient is lying on the operation table, whether it is an ISAF colleague, a local, an Afghan soldier or even an enemy fighter. Even the people who wouldn't think twice about blowing us up, are being helped. I am livid about this and on top of that I have also noticed a different sort of anger rise inside of me.

Why hasn't there been more focus on the threat during our preparation? If the missile attacks are such a well-known phenomenon, like that Englishman said to us when we arrived, why weren't we informed properly? Why wasn't it mentioned that it can completely change your perception of everything?

What stayed with me most of the entire prep course are the stories about how some people can cheaply sort out a stable internet connection for you at Kandahar Airfield. And that it is possible to ship genuine Persian rugs to home. And of course that there are a couple of fast-food chains trucks along the boardwalk. The ideal solution for a quick bite. And not to forget: the *iced frappuccino* of coffee chain Tim Hortons, possibly the best in the world. These were the most important bits of information that I picked up.

There has definitely not been sufficient focus on the ever-present threat, let alone on what it can actually do to people. I think the impact that a war, the threat and war victims can have on someone, isn't emphasised enough.

I have only just arrived at work this morning when a bright laugh sounds through the hospital. On the ward, little Aziz is having fun on a children's bike. Laughing out loud, Aziz bikes through the hospital. I stop to look at him and just like many others in the hospital I smile. He sits on the bike in a t-shirt that is way too big for him and he is wearing brand-new sandals, whilst his father, who walks next to him in a typical dress and pair of trousers, is wearing old sandals. He puts his hand on his son's shoulder when he notices that people, me included, are watching them. Then they both smile.

It is a good sign that Aziz is out of bed. Under guidance of a nurse he bikes out of the hospital. The basket on the handlebars carries a syringe, filled with medication. Even though he still looks very poorly, there is a giant smile on his gaunt little face.

Seeing Aziz like this makes me feel happy. A smiling patient with his proud and grateful father. Sometimes things do go right.

The next child at our hospital would leave a completely different impression.

The day starts in a surprising way when we report to the hospital. A few Canadian and American citizens are walking around. Journalists, photographers and one of them is a so-called *war artist*. He follows us for a day with a camera around his neck. He creates beautiful black and white sketches from all the pictures he takes. A true artist. After having witnessed a couple of procedures he tells me that he is also moved by everything he witnesses, the ugly face of war.

The summer has well and truly started in southern Afghanistan. Today is the hottest day of my entire deployment. In the afternoon the thermometer reads 63.9 degrees Celsius. It hurts to walk outside.

Sitting in the shade, I drink one bottle of water after another. The heat makes me almost long for a notification from the hospital, so we can go to the cool operating room where it is only 30 degrees Celsius. It sounds positively refreshing. It only takes a short while before my unspoken wish is granted.

The alert concerns an Afghan police officer who got injured in an explosion and is already on his way by helicopter.

He is admitted to hospital in the usual way, is stabilised and then taken into the operating room. The wounds on his legs, arms and shoulders are cleaned and bandaged. There is nothing remarkable about the procedure, other than the photographers who are swarming us like flies around shit. Their cameras are clicking constantly. A couple of days later there would be pictures on the internet with the headline stating that Dutch and Canadian medics work together like a band of brothers.

I didn't know then, that later that day I would get really angry with that same clicking. I couldn't have suspected that I would be really moved and extremely annoyed too.

That night we are told about an injured and seriously ill child who will be brought from the Mirwais hospital. The local doctors simply don't know what to do with the boy who was shot in his abdomen and upper leg a few days ago. The leg doesn't look good and his health is deteriorating. We are asked to get the operating room ready.

When he is brought in we see a 12-year-old boy and he looks terrible. Tubes are draining fluids from multiple places in his abdomen. The right leg is covered by a sheet.

We remove it from his leg after we have laid him down on the operating table. Then I see the damage and I can't breathe for a moment. What the hell happened here? His leg has been cut open in several places. There are long incisions on the lower and upper leg. It has been opened up down to the muscle layers, but the muscular tissue isn't a healthy red, but rather a discoloured dark and grey. The whole leg is swollen, from the groin down to the toes. A bluish shiny glow can be seen all over the limb. It has obviously started to die.

The orthopaedic surgeon begins to explain. This boy was taken into surgery in Mirwais soon after he was shot. The doctors there were not able to control the bleeding in his groin. To stem the flow of blood they eventually ligated the veins. That is where something has gone horribly wrong. At first glance, the veins as well as the femoral artery seem to have been tied off. This main artery provides oxygen to the leg and by tying it off, the leg has been deprived of it. This has naturally caused the leg to start dying and that process is now irreversible.

We have to prepare ourselves for an amputation of this boy's whole leg. That is, if he stays alive, as he really is seriously ill. First, we will need to open his abdomen because the surgeon wants to check whether there is a problem that the Afghan doctors might have missed.

"If only a few miles away they tie off a femoral artery like this, then it's worth having a look to see what they were up to in his abdomen," the surgeon says cynically.

I notice that everyone is distraught once they have seen the child. It all seems so senseless. If he would have ended up on our operating table straight after he was shot, we most certainly could have saved his leg. Then he wouldn't have had to be so ill. With the right intensive care, he would not have suffered this much.

I quickly share some thoughts with our anaesthetist and he tells me that the child's kidneys are badly affected.

"It'll be an almighty miracle if he survives."

We will probably succeed in making sure this patient leaves our table alive but the period directly after the surgery, at the intensive care ward, will be tense. He will occupy one of the beds for a long time and everyone will be fighting for his life.

"Damn, Linda," I say, "this little dude had all the luck in the world to get to that hospital in Mirwais alive. And then it is as if they do all they can to not help him survive."

What sort of doctors work there? How stupid can you be to tie off a pulsing artery that is as wide as a thumb and subsequently be surprised that the leg starts to stink and die. First they nearly let the child die to then ring those 'western dogs' of ISAF at the last possible moment to see if they can help. And what will the result be? We will again amputate a leg of a young child. A child who, because of us, will be sentenced to a life full of worries.

When I think of the degree of care and empathy in this country, I don't foresee a lot of good for him. It annoys me immensely and I feel an anger in myself that I can hardly control.

At exactly that moment I am pushed away by a photographer. Armed with an expensive camera he wants to take a few detailed pictures of the leg. I step aside for a minute. I then ask my colleague if she has prepared everything for the procedure. She has. I can now focus on positioning the patient and disinfecting the abdomen and leg.

I hear the constant clicking of cameras all around me. The operating room is filled to the rafters with people who all want to take a pic of this 'interesting case'. After I have been pushed aside a few times my stress levels have reached boiling point. With an ice-cold voice I ask them to leave theatre. A child is dying here and he needs immediate surgical care. Their reactions are too slow for my liking.

"Everyone who isn't directly involved in this operation needs to get lost now! Get the fuck out!" I shout across the room. I am fuming and put all my venom in that one sentence. Am I really angry with them, or am I furious because of this poor child? He should be playing outside, or be helping with dinner. He should definitely not be the victim of gunfire.

People look at me bewildered. Obviously, they did not see that coming. One by one the paparazzi leave the room. After my outburst it is completely silent for a moment, except for the beeps of the anaesthesia equipment.

Everybody talks quietly. The surgery's aim is explained briefly. First the abdomen will be opened to have a closer look at it. Once possible injuries have been taken care of, we will continue with the leg that will be amputated from the hip joint, a so-called *disarticulation*. This means that the whole leg under the buttock will be removed. Because of this there is little hope that a prosthesis will actually fit. This type of advanced prosthetics is probably not available here. But the first challenge will be to help this child live through these tough operations.

The surgery on the abdomen goes smoothly. The abdominal cavity and the organs are inspected and flushed. It is then neatly closed. As soon as the wound is bandaged, we move on to prepare the child for the final, invasive and awfully maiming operation.

The surgeon starts the amputation with stern efficiency. The procedure can be described as a massacre. All surgical drapes covering the patient quickly turn a deep red. There are several puddles of blood under the operating table.

The sickly scent of rotting flesh spreads through theatre. The surgeons work through all structures in a short space of time. At some stage I notice one of them working on the groin. Silently he passes Linda a piece of tissue. She takes it and when she looks at it I can see her bewilderment. Her eyes meet mine. On the gauze in her bloodstained surgical glove is a testicle of the boy.

Dismayed she throws the gauze with the tissue in the red bin bag I have opened for her. The specialists continue to work silently and calmly and after a while ask for the saw. The leg is sawn off just under the head of the femur.

I wait with the red rubbish bag in my hands. The surgeon signals at me to open it. Blood from the freshly amputated leg gushes over my gloves. He carefully slides the whole leg into the bag, but it is too big to fit properly. Only after a bit of swearing and shaking the leg fits in the bag. I write the patient number on a label and attach it. Then I start my walk to the white refrigerated container as I don't want to keep this leg in my OR for another minute.

I struggle more each time I step into that container and it is particularly difficult to simply throw away a part of a child. Inside I hold my breath and I put the bag around the corner to the right with a big pile of other bags. Then I turn around to step outside again. I trip and because of that I forget to hold my breath. I gag when the smell reaches my brain and I fall flat on my stomach. I kick against whatever it was that tripped me up. The dull, soggy sound makes me think it is a leg. I wryly note that I nearly got tackled by an amputated leg. I lock the container and hurry back to theatre.

They are still working hard to close the huge wound. This all happens with the efficiency of a well-oiled machine. The stump is taken care of and bandaged in the best possible way. A bit later I add the last details to the surgical report and notice that these two procedures have altogether taken less than two hours. That is all it took to change this boy's life dramatically.

One hundred and twenty minutes that would resonate with me for a long time: my outburst at the photographers, the miserable sight, the nauseating smell and the noises when I put the young, amputated leg in the corner of the container. This boy is one of those patients I will never forget.

I wonder why I am so agitated. Is it because of the helplessness I feel? This child didn't receive the care it should have received. Or is it because of something else?

The image of the boy on the operating table, with us like a bunch of butchers, moves me. We operate on his abdomen, amputate an entire leg, and casually remove a testicle. Another happy patient, I think cynically.

What has raised doubts before, but bothers me more each day, is what actually happens to the patients after our intervention. Take this child. What if he survives? Our colleagues at the intensive care will do all they can to keep this child alive. And then what? This boy will probably have to go and beg, or will have to be taken care of by his family. Will this happen, or will he be rejected?

$\sim$

It is late in the evening when I sit in my sleeping quarters. I can't shake off the image of the child. It gets to me to see a little body shot to pieces.

I phone home straight after we finish helping the boy. I need to hear my sons. It is wonderful to hear their cheerful and bright voices. I tell them how happy I am with their beautiful drawings and encourage them to make more.

"Daddy, the sweetie jar doesn't seem to get less full at all." My eldest son couldn't have said it better.

THE BUCKET FILLS UP

The last couple of days the camp has been shot at more than once per day. Today is no different.

A huge blast shakes the ground. A couple of seconds later the wailing of sirens swells.

"Rocket attack, rocket attack."

The tinny female voice echoes through loudspeakers all around camp. Again, we drop what we are doing and fall to the floor. After a while we run to the nearest bunker, because it never stops at one blast. We wait for the next one and don't have to wait long.

I was absolutely terrified the first time I experienced a missile hitting our base. So many would follow that I am used to it now. I do sometimes wonder, whilst I am in the bunker, how much longer this will go on for? Until now no one has been hurt by the attacks, but will there come a time when the missile does serious damage? I can't seem to relax anymore. I have worked at this heavily guarded base that is regularly hit by missile attacks for weeks. Even though it seems to be equipped with many facilities, it is still right in the middle of a war-stricken country where we are faced with the worst facets of warfare every day.

Some days I despise the fact that I assist with procedures that change a patient's life so dramatically. That feeling increases during my deployment.

"I think the worst thing that could happen to a patient is surviving," I often say out loud to myself and to my colleagues. We help patients from all walks of life. From coalition soldiers of ISAF, but also the ANA military, the ANP police officers to the civilian population; and even enemy fighters too, the so-called OMF, *Opposing Militant Forces*, or Taliban. So, we even take care of the enemy who detests everything we stand for. In accordance with laws, regulations and ethics every person is entitled to help, without exception and of course we comply with these rules.

During the last part of my deployment a couple of things would happen in quick succession that hit me hard. They would make me feel helpless, deprive me of my pride and destroy my self-image.

HAPPY BIRTHDAY TO YOU

"Oh yes, the damn progress in this fucking country is so obvious! A woman's position hasn't improved one bit here! Look there, proof! Oh, we do such meaningful work!" I spit out my words. I express all the sarcasm and venom I feel.

My colleague, who has joined me as I walk around the field, looks at me for a moment. He doesn't respond. He closely studies the ground in front of his feet as we walk on in silence. I wipe the sweat off my forehead, while my gaze stays focused on the scene just outside the gates.

About 200 feet away from the field are a couple of houses, flats, partially shot to pieces. They are still occupied though. On the top floor is a home which hardly has a front wall left. There is washing drying up there. It looks like someone is walking through the house.

A woman walks alone on the deserted road in front of the flat. She is completely covered in a blue burqa. It is a haunting image. The surroundings are desolate. Everywhere I look, I see a lifeless grey. The woman dressed in her bright blue robe stands out from this grey scene.

There are lots of these burqas for sale at the bazaar on the base and people joke about them. Now I am actually confronted with a woman dressed like this, I can't think of a bad joke at all. I pity her, and everything I do here suddenly seems so very pointless. My armour is starting to crack.

The last couple of days have been much increasingly busy in the hospital. We perform lots of surgeries, not only during shifts, but also on our days off. As soon as the daily stream of patients starts, the decision is made to page the second surgical team too. Some days that is not even enough, which is why both teams regularly operate deep into the night.

As the surgery days in hospital get longer, our sleep gets shorter. I try to rest whenever possible and I often isolate myself to lie down on my bed for an hour. I feel better on my own. The tension isn't only increasing in the hospital, but also in my head. Slowly but surely, I am feeling numb to most patients and their injuries.

The atmosphere in the OR and in our team is changing gradually. People snap at each other and here and there small annoyances are building. It is obviously getting tense for others too.

As ever, I try not to show that I am struggling. During the day I put on my happiest mask, but meanwhile my sense of humour is getting harsher and darker. It is my way of laughing off the misery. Everything I thought was interesting and new during the first couple of weeks, is now completely normal. I am annoyed by everyone and everything and not in the least by myself.

During that week I decide that I am going to resign from the army as soon as possible after my deployment. It is time to return to civilian life as I don't want to be sent to another country where barbarity rules.

~

The right leg of the police officer on the operating table has been maimed beyond recognition. The X-rays show what the explosion has done to the internal parts of the leg. This is going to be a tough job. The left leg is positioned in an unnatural angle, but at least it looks like it can be saved.

The man drove over a roadside bomb in his car. Apart from the injuries to his leg, his eye has also been severely damaged. A fragment entered and has caused irreparable damage.

We start surgery on both legs. During the procedure we are standing in a large puddle of blood. The specialists try to save the patient's right leg, but it is a lost cause. There is an almost palpable motivation to save the other leg. It takes hours, but at least we are able to save his left leg.

Eye surgery is next. The injury is so severe that it has been decided to remove the eye before the procedure even starts. Prior to this surgery, the surgeon has already made several little balls of bone cement, in different sizes, and has had them sterilised.

We will use one to fill up the eye cavity, once the eye has been removed. Eye prosthetics aren't available here and it is and always will be a case of improvising.

Some hours after he was brought in severely injured, the policeman leaves the operating table with one less leg and one less eye. He has been given a ball of cement instead. Not the best of swaps.

History teaches us that lots of medical discoveries and developments have happened during wartime. I experience that first-hand. Somehow, we have to treat all wounded who arrive on our operating table with limited resources. Sometimes we start with just a scalpel and go along with what we find. On the one hand this a beautiful way of working as it requires a lot of creativity and resourcefulness. On the other hand it is too depressing to even think about, because we can't offer care at the level of a well-equipped hospital.

A very special surgery, during which creativity will play a big part, is coming up. A police officer has been brought in with multiple injuries. Other than a femur fracture, that will be stabilised with a pin, he also has a major injury to his hand.

"Hey, he actually has a hole in his hand," I say looking at his injury.

There is a gaping hole through both the palm and the back of his hand. It is such a serious injury that I expect him to leave the table without a hand.

"Easy one, that'll come off, we'll be done nice and early." I say this out loud as I get the red waste bag ready. Nothing could be further from the truth. Even though it is the left hand, which is considered to be unclean, we will still do everything we can to save it.

Once the operation on his fractured right leg is finished, we prepare the hand for surgery. As soon as the patient is completely covered with surgical drapes I look once more from the hand to the X-rays and back again. I sigh and get to work.

"Scalpel," the surgeon says.

I pass the scalpel and then we start.

The bullet went right through his hand. On its way through, it completely destroyed the metacarpals of the middle and ring finger. The plan is to end up with a partly functioning hand.

The orthopaedic surgeon explains how he wants to achieve that. The middle finger, ring finger, and the underlying ruined metacarpals will be removed. Both fingers won't be removed in full though, they will be stripped. The little joints will be taken out, while the skin remains attached to the hand. The skin of the fingers will be used at the end of surgery to cover big holes. His hand will be narrowed when all joints and metacarpals have been removed. This means his little finger will be next to the index finger.

After operating for a while both his fingers have been completely stripped of the skin and can be amputated. The fingers with three phalanxes, connected by ligaments, are passed to me.

"Look Linda, they still work, this is awesome!" Triumphantly I hold a finger up in the air in front of me and shake it a couple of times. The finger, though without any skin, moves as if it makes a 'come here' movement. Some people chuckle.

With a careless gesture I throw both fingers in the red bag. The chuckling immediately silences.

During the hours that follow I assist in the recovery operation. The hand is narrowed, the little finger is positioned in its new place and the large wounds are closed. After all the wounds are closed, a little claw is all that is left. It resembles a chicken leg. It is a technical masterpiece, but it doesn't make me happy.

I have had enough of it all but will have to keep going for a bit longer. There happens to be another patient straight away. This one has multiple bullet wounds too, which need immediate attention. This procedure takes several hours and it is nearly night when I leave the hospital.

Food is arranged for us on the days that we simply can not leave the operating room during the day. In a tent behind the hospital are trays full of whatever is on the menu. These look like feeding troughs. On the days that I hear dinner is served and that I can go and eat, I always, while running out of the operating room, shout that 'I am going to stick my snout in the trough'. The others grin. The role of joker, the one that makes others smile, suits me. It is a role I have taken on at the expense of myself. But today we are done on time, so instead of the lukewarm grub from the trough I am able to eat a decent meal in the dining hall. I enjoy it to the fullest.

When I am off work, I lie on my bed a lot, listen to music and write letters home. I try to ring home as much as possible. Although it is nice to hear the voices of my wife and my kids, it is extremely frustrating to not be able to say how I really feel.

The last days of July have now begun and the pressure on my body and spirit is increasing with every tough operation we do. I notice that on the one hand I am becoming insensitive to most injuries and the people behind them. On the other hand, some patients, like children, hit me like a sledgehammer. It hurts and makes me realise I want to go home, to my family and I want to turn this black page of the book called my life as quickly as possible. I would rather tear it out and throw it away, so I never have to look at it again.

With this month nearing its end, my youngest son's birthday is also coming closer. I have bought a pile of toys in the American tax-free shop. It is a strange experience to walk into a shop on a huge military base in the middle of a war zone, and to be able to buy whatever I want. From widescreen televisions to bicycles. I hope that the Lego arrives on time, so that he still gets a present from his daddy from faraway Afghanistan. I would love to be there for his special day to blow out the candles together, but instead, we welcome back an old acquaintance on our operating table.

Just before the birthday I am more irritable than normal. I don't think it is simply because I miss my home front. During that warm month of July in the desert I increasingly struggle with the injuries that people here inflict upon each other. I also struggle with my own stubbornness, as I don't want to discuss it. I recognise it, as I have been doing it like this for years: don't talk about anything and keep on going.

That is exactly what I do after a long night when I kick open the backdoor of the hospital to take the rubbish bags to the white container. As soon as I step outside I am confronted with four dead Afghan soldiers. Their still uncovered bodies are on stretchers. They are victims of yet another attack or gunfight. I stride past them and glance back at them one more time to then continue with my task, but the image doesn't leave me. The heads of the dead droop backwards or sideways. A couple of them still have their eyes open. The arms are next to the body. The outerwear of two of the men has been cut open and evidence of rescue attempts can be seen on their bare torsos. The other two are still completely dressed in uniform and in multiple places their fatigues are coloured red.

Why is this image getting to me so much, I wonder. Aren't they just another bunch of deceased Afghan soldiers? Is it because I stepped into the dark and was confronted by death? I walk back to the hospital after getting rid of the waste. I don't tell anyone about the deceased soldiers and what it did to me. Once again I hold back the words I want to say.

A little later I sit on my bed and out of the blue I start to cry. Tears are streaming down my face. Immediately after, I have a long and emotional chat with Linda. I tell her that I have spent years not talking about things and that I always set the bar high. I do that for others, but that bar is set even higher for myself. We talk for a long time. Although I don't tell her very many facts, I do tell her who I really am. For the very first time I take off my mask and show the person that has been hiding behind it. The one that is always there for others, but completely neglects himself in the meantime. The burden I have been carrying for much too long glides off my shoulders. I have been such a good clown. Professionally I still consider this mission to be the most interesting period of my career. I keep trying to make the best of it and I try to keep smiling. I don't do that to entertain others, but to keep myself going. I really hope I can keep it up.

On the 30th of July I wake up from a restless sleep.

"Happy birthday to you, I wish I was home with you," I sing out loud when I get out of bed.

Today is the birthday of my youngest son Lars. I am gutted I am not there to enjoy it with him. I curse the fact I am here.

As I am smoking my first cigarette of the day I think about some of the victims we have seen so far. I conclude that every day seems to get harder for me. Especially the kids affect me. Some are hurt by war violence, others by sheer bad luck or domestic violence. They make me want to go home.

Today we welcome back an old acquaintance to our table. The high-ranking patient who had major injury to his left arm will undergo his corrective surgery. I thought his arm would have to be amputated, but I was wrong. We are going to correct the bone defect in his forearm, by implanting a part of the fibula.

I am still astounded by the surgical possibilities under these far from ideal circumstances. The huge lack of hygiene, the ever-present dust, but also the few negative consequences they apparently have. I again wonder if this is because people here have a much higher resistance, or because we worry too much about hygiene and infections in the western world.

The procedure takes a couple of hours and goes without complications. It looks like this is going to be a patient who we have actually been able to help. Despite the success rate of the procedure I am in a foul mood for the rest of the day. My thoughts are with my birthday boy and the rest of my family.

I warn everybody that I am insufferable today, and that I am not in the mood for drivel. I grab a black marker pen and in big letters I write 'Go Away!!!' on the back of my surgical top.

With a surly face I stomp through the hospital on my clogs. Again, everyone chuckles at the sight of me and the text on my back. I hear many times today that I am a great joker and that I positively influence the mood. It is a dubious honour.

REPATRIATION

I chuck the end of my fag onto the concrete of the platform. I am dressed in green scrubs and have my bright yellow clogs on my feet. A surgical cap with a cherry pattern sits on my head. The clogs make a scraping noise over the concrete when I stamp out the smouldering cigarette end. Then I pick it up and pop it in the small breast pocket of my scrub shirt.

It is the middle of the night and we have just finished surgery on some severely wounded victims. We have spent the entire day in the operating room. Another day with injured and maimed patients. It just doesn't seem to end.

A quick calculation in my head tells me we have performed surgery for nearly 18 hours today. It feels like I have been here for years, but in reality it has only been several weeks. I am not even halfway through my assignment. Well, at least we haven't lost any patients today.

The platform with the enormous plane is covered in darkness. The only visible light comes from the aircraft. The ramp at the back has been lowered. People are preparing for the evacuation of some wounded American soldiers.

High above I can hear an annoying buzz. It is as if a swarm of wasps is lurking somewhere. It is probably the Predator UAV, an *unmanned aerial vehicle*, otherwise known as a *drone*. A few of those devices are stationed here at Kandahar Airfield.

I wonder if the person who operates it, from a safe control room somewhere in the United States, is looking in on what is about to happen here. Or perhaps this drone is equipped with a heavy bomb, and has taken off to hunt for enemy fighters or other suspicious people, who are somewhere in the more inhospitable areas of Afghanistan? If that is the case, this UAV will give those folks a particularly bad day today. Their last one.

From a distance, six ambulances are approaching. Their lights are dimmed. They stop close to the open ramp of the aircraft. With military precision the ambulances are parked so that the nurses only need to walk a short distance to carry the poor souls onto the plane. One by one the victims are offloaded from the cars to then disappear into the plane as fast as they have arrived.

The belly of the huge C-17 Globemaster III, the Cadillac of transport planes, is hungry today. No less than nine wounded American soldiers are gobbled up. They are being evacuated to Germany to receive further treatment. For now, they have been stabilised and have had necessary life-saving surgery here at Role 3.

The injured are stable enough to make the long trip to Germany to begin their recovery. It will be a long journey for them, the road home as well as the road to recovery, as far as that is even possible.

They are welcomed on the plane with the greatest of respect. I see how the nurses talk to some the victims and notice one of the injured crying uncontrollably. The nurse who is looking after him, puts his hand on the shoulder of the sobbing lad, as he is assigned a place on the aircraft. I am not sure whether he is crying because of the nature of his injuries or because it feels wrong for him to leave his unit.

When the last of the wounded is carried onto the plane the ambulances disappear again. It doesn't take long before the ramp is closed. I stay where I am on the taxiway, where two colleagues have now joined me. All three of us light a cigarette in silence.

When the plane rolls past, we raise our hand to the pilots. In the dim light of the instruments in the cockpit we notice the crew waving back at us. The bulky airplane passes us by and makes its way onto the long taxiway to the start of the runway.

The men who have just been carried onto the plane have to prepare for a whole new type of battle. A few of them looked in really bad shape. They were more dead than alive.

A dirty and dastardly battle rages only a few miles from here. A guerrilla war in which Afghan police officers and soldiers, coalition forces and civilians are wounded and killed every day.

The young men and women of the coalition forces, who exit the base daily to go on patrol, are aware of it. They hope every single day that they will return safely that night, with all their limbs there where they belong.

"Sleep for a bit, Erik, try and rest. It's been another busy one today. At least the guys on the plane made it."

My two colleagues watch the plane disappear from sight on the taxiway. I nod and smoke a bit more. It is always impressive to see that such a giant can actually take off at all.

I put my fingers in my ears, as the plane's engines are now going at full force and the heavy C-17 starts to move. It hurls past, the nose goes up and the aircraft soon comes off the ground. It starts to climb and quickly disappears into the night.

CREATIVE AND INVENTIVE PATCHWORK

It is so confrontational. A child whose entire leg had to be amputated is coming back today for a follow-up operation. The stump has to be opened up and cleaned.

As he is being brought in on a stretcher an old man follows right behind him. I am not sure if he is the father or another family member. We lift the child from the stretcher onto the operating table and cover him up with blankets. The old man stays close to him.

I am in the back of the operating room and help Linda by passing the sterile equipment. At the same time we watch the man who is waiting with the boy. When he sees us looking at him, he gives us an almost toothless smile. He places his hand on his heart and bows slightly.

Did I see that right? Is it a sign of appreciation or gratitude? I can hardly believe it. Is it really true that I am looking at a man who is grateful that his family member is still alive? Despite the fact that we, as 'infidels', have amputated this child's leg and therefore made him useless as a breadwinner, the man actually seems to be truly grateful for the boy's life.

Clumsily I also make a little bow, after which I quickly turn around and pretend to be very busy with something really important. The man's small gesture triggers a whole range of emotions. I am moved by it and this would become the trend for the following weeks. As the work pressure increases, my resilience seems to be crumbling. The professional distance I always used to keep between me and my patients has slowly started to break down.

~

"Erik, we lost a patient. You guys have just performed surgery on him, but now he's gone."

I warily look at the anaesthetist as I stop mopping the floor of the operating theatre for a moment. I give him an obvious answer.

"Eh? That's not possible."

It is a patient whose jaw was shot to pieces, which we reconstructed with screws and plates. After that procedure we fixated his mandibular with steel wires to the upper jaw. It will need to stay like that for a couple of weeks. He will have to eat liquidised food and he will need to carry a heavy-duty pair of scissors with him at all times in case he has to vomit. The steel wires can then be cut loose to prevent him choking on his own vomit. It can't be possible that this patient has walked out of the hospital just like that.

Just to be sure, I walk to the back of the hospital and to my surprise I find the patient there. He is standing in the sunshine, smoking a cigarette with his wired jaws. He looks like it is the most natural thing of the world and smiles broadly to expose his wire fencing as I wildly gesture for him to get inside.

I can't help it, but it makes me laugh. I call inside to let them know that I have found the patient and that I will bring him back. But not before we have both smoked a cigarette with big smiles on our faces.

It proves to be one of our longer days. We work till deep into the night on a couple of Afghan soldiers who were ambushed. The final patient surprises me. He has bullet wounds in his foot and his hand. This soldier got hurt during a fight with his own colleagues, as they stopped him from killing himself. We are going to fix someone who wanted to end it all, which I incidentally can imagine amidst all of this misery.

First of all we are going to do a hand narrowing procedure on this patient and then we will place some screws in his foot.

As far as I know an attempted suicide is a great sin in this culture. Those that commit it will be punished. It won't surprise me if this guy will still be killed after we have helped him. It makes me annoyed to think that we might be sacrificing our time and resources on someone who will probably die anyway. We do this so the patient can walk out of the hospital to then be handed over to the authorities. They will probably finish what the patient initially started and wanted. A waste of time and materials. I don't get it at all.

The days go by in a haze and it is getting busier by the day. We are often working till deep into the night. Where I meticulously kept track of everything I experienced, saw and felt during the first weeks of my deployment, I only see a few notes in my diary for the month of August. Even nice things I experienced, have been snowed under in a pool of misery.

There are signs that I am not the only one for whom the pressure is building steadily. Angry words are thrown back and forth within our team during the umpteenth surgery day with multiple injured who were all brought in simultaneously.

The atmosphere in the team has changed after the outburst.

I feel miserable that this has happened. I always felt secure amidst my team members, but now that too has changed. Together we have to try and make it work for another couple of weeks. They will be very long weeks indeed. But thank goodness the end is in sight.

There is a lot of talk about our departure from Kandahar. We feel that a decompression period in Crete would be beneficial to us, but after enquiring over and over again we are told that these adaptation days still haven't been organised. A small team like ours, that wasn't flown out at the same time with the big deployment rotation, won't be flown into Crete on its own.

Up to the last week of our deployment we are unsure about the schedule of our return journey and we don't know when and via where we will be flying back. During this uncertain time I am so pleased I put more sweets in the jar for the boys. It is better to be safe than sorry.

Eventually, after asking over and over again, we are informed we will definitely not be flying home via Crete. Via a military base in the United Arab Emirates we will fly directly to Amsterdam. There won't be a heartwarming return to our military airfield where friends and family would be waiting for us. We will be flying home anonymously on a charter flight and travel amongst holidaymakers.

"It is a monster," I stammer.

As soon as the patient arrives in the operating room, I look into the saddest pair of eyes I have ever seen. They catch my eye and pierce my soul. Pain shoots through my heart and nestles itself deep within my core. I am deeply moved by the sight of this young man. The young Afghan soldier we are operating had surgery on his bottom jaw a couple of weeks ago in this very same hospital. Today I see the impact of war surgery. Instead of being brought in on a stretcher, the proud young man walks into the OR on his own. He climbs onto the operating table independently and lies down. His frightened eyes dart from left to right.

His mouth stands at an odd angle. He wheezes and the interpreter is struggling to communicate with him. The X-rays show a seemingly well-constructed jaw, but it matches in no way with what I am looking at here.

I see a young man who has difficulty breathing. Talking is virtually impossible for him, because his tongue hardly functions. The interpreter explains to us that eating and drinking is a true ordeal for this young man, and only really works when food is placed in the back of his mouth, so all he needs to do is swallow. And even swallowing is like top sport to him.

We are going to perform a reconstruction, with the aim of lessening some of the limitations, so that he can function better and meet his basic needs. How many patients who need more treatment after our patching up will actually be seen again? The man who is on our table now has been lucky to be able to come back. Hopefully we can offer him a better quality of life.

It is a routine operation, however at the end of the procedure I have no idea what we have actually improved. The surgeon seems satisfied though. I am holding on to the fact that we have brought some relief to the patient, but I can't be sure.

The look in his eyes, the sadness and the helplessness really get to me. Although this patient has definitely not got the worst acute injuries I have seen here, he has still moved me deeply. What are the consequences of our surgical intervention?

I would ask that same question after the next procedure. An older Taliban fighter has been admitted to hospital. The ball of his left upper arm has been shot to smithereens.

Even though he is the enemy, it is decided that we will do our utmost to save the arm. To do so we have found a creative solution. A pin that would normally be used for a small child with a femur fracture is being manually adapted. New drill holes are being added to the pin in several places, after which it is sterilised, so that it can be inserted backwards to save the arm.

We perform another technical and inventive masterpiece. This procedure is successful too and the customised solution means that the patient is able to keep his arm. All the X-rays show our brilliant solution and everybody seems very impressed by what we just did.

After the surgery I think again about the young soldier from days ago. The big difference between him and our last patient is that I only stop and think about today's patient for a moment. This is partly because I see something else in him, as he embodies the cause of the injuries of all other patients we see here and I don't feel anything when I think about him. To put it even more strongly, somewhere in the back of my head is a voice that whispers softly that I hope that this patient will leave the hospital with his arm. But I also hope that it will function as badly as the bottom jaw of that poor young soldier. I hope the arm will be like a dead weight.

It is absolutely not ethically right or politically correct to think this, but Afghanistan is not particularly known for being politically correct itself. I have seen too many examples of this over the past weeks.

We don't see the man again after the surgery. He is being nursed in a separate room with a 24-hour guard in front of the door.

To this day I still have no clue how he left the hospital. Whether he was handed over the local authorities, and what actually happened to him and his arm, I have no idea and I couldn't care less.

$\sim$

"Erik, when was the last time you assisted with brain surgery?" the orthopaedic surgeon asks me.

I have to think about that for a while. "Well, years ago I had an internship at the neurosurgery department of a university hospital and observed those sorts of procedures, but I have never actually assisted with one," is my answer.

"Perfect, a wealth of experience then. Ha, you're almost overqualified!," the surgeon jokes after which he tells me I can help him.

We will be performing surgery on an Afghan soldier who has suffered a bullet wound to his head.

A little later I am assisting with the procedure. After a lot of to-ing and fro-ing we have been able to position the patient on the operating table so we can open the cranium. In the absence of a neurosurgeon, the orthopaedic surgeon and the maxillofacial surgeon will perform the surgery together.

From what I understand the surgeons will mainly remove metal particles and loose bone fragments from the patient's head. When I hear that we are done after operating for a long time, I once again get the feeling that I have helped with something of which the outcome is not quite clear. It mirrors the overall feeling I now have about our work in the hospital. It is makeshift. It is making do. Quality of life seems to be less important. We reach our goal when patients leave our table with a beating heart. That seems to be the mantra I hold on to. I am here to save lives, and that is what we do. We are providing 'the best care anywhere', under the given circumstances. Slowly but surely I get swept away by this thought. It feels as though my empathy towards patients is slowly decreasing. I have started to feel numb most of the time.

There are still those rare moments when we have a patient who opens my eyes and gets to me though. It is usually in a negative way, but once in a while something happens that leaves a positive impression. Something that makes me happy. Something that doesn't show the destruction of human life, but the complete opposite.

NEW LIFE

There is peace and quiet at the hospital. After peak voltage the pressure cooker only has the little pilot light on today.

We are notified of three casualties late in the afternoon. Two Afghan soldiers and one civilian were injured during a firefight. The soldiers both have a femur fracture as a result of gunfire. The third patient is an Afghan woman. She has also been hit by a bullet. It has drilled its way through her jaw. Her headscarf is wet and dark with blood. It promises to be another late night. When I look the woman in the eye, I sense there is something else. Only when I look at the noticeboard in the corridor, I read that she is about eight months pregnant. How sad, that such a vulnerable woman is struck by war violence.

The Canadian surgical team has also been called in. They will be taking care of her, while we operate the two wounded soldiers. Both procedures go as planned. The fractures are stabilised with a pin in the femur and the woman's bottom jaw is reconstructed with plates and screws. The operations are considered to be a success.

I suddenly see the young Afghan soldier with the sad look in his eyes before me again. I hope that the pregnant woman won't be inconvenienced too much by what she has been through, war violence and our actions alike.

$$\sim$$

It is already near midnight and we are still working on the second injured soldier. Our colleagues in the other operating room have now finished reconstructing the woman's jaw.

There is new patient though, this time a very young patient indeed as the woman is about to give birth. This causes quite some commotion, nearly panic, in the hospital. The Role 3 is equipped to take care of war victims, but gynaecology and obstetrics are not specialisms we cover here. This hospital isn't prepared for childbirth at all. Where do we get a crib and where do we get an incubator? Our colleagues are in uproar whilst we still sort out the soldier's femur fracture. Various nurses try and find items to make sure the baby will be delivered safely.

When we lift the soldier from the operating table, we get the message that the woman has just given birth to a healthy baby boy. A wave of relaxation engulfs the hospital. A little later the psychiatrist is parading through the hospital with a baby in his arms and I see smiling faces everywhere. He shows us the baby too. It is a moving sight. Finally, an event in this horrific place that has nothing to do with the mutilation and destruction of life, but with the start of a new one.

A hard rock song about the birth of a child is blasting from the CD player in the OR. I see multiple people with tears in their eyes. My lip starts to tremble too, but quickly I man up.

Later that night in bed I wonder what will become of the newborn. Will his mum tell him later that he was delivered by a group of western infidels? Will they be grateful? It all seems so pointless and ambiguous. It feels fantastic to be present at the start of a new life, but at the same time I wonder if this little man is a budding bomber. Shocked, I realise that I already identify this innocent little being with this country's evil.

AN EXTRA HAND

Amidst all the misery sometimes there is a day that stays with me in a really positive way.

I meet Peter right at the beginning of my deployment. He is a weapons engineer in the Airforce and a very warm guy I regularly meet up with on base. He is always up for a cup of coffee and a good chat. We decide that it would be interesting to have a look at each other's work for half a day. He takes me for a tour of his workplace and we have a really enjoyable day. When it is my turn I invite him to come and have a look in the hospital and I tell him to have a hearty breakfast that morning.

It is nothing new to have spectators in our operating room. We quickly arrange a date for him and two of his colleagues. A few days later Peter walks into the hospital to observe a surgery.

We have a patient with a bullet wound to his abdomen. It has damaged the colon and we will remove that part. After a short talk with the surgeon I invite Peter to come over to the operating table under my guidance, so he can be as close as possible. Peter changes into scrubs. I help him with his sterile gown and the sterile surgical gloves. The transformation is complete.

Dressed as a true operating room nurse, Peter is allowed to join us at the table. It proves to be an amazing experience for all of us. The surgery goes smoothly and the surgeon does everything he can to explain to our guest what we are doing. And Peter? He is noticeably enjoying himself and talks non-stop in his own dry, humorous way. He gets everyone laughing and by doing that he actually assists with surgery. It is a morning in a million.

An abdomen surgery and a good vibe in the operation room. It actually feels like a regular workday. Afterwards Peter helps to tidy up. When it is all done we sit in the bunker behind the hospital and discuss the morning, accompanied by a bottle of water and tough stories. I am really enjoying myself and for a while I forget everything around me.

A FRESH (HEAD)WIND

A new Canadian unit has recently taken over the command of the hospital.

Everywhere I look I see pale faces, not yet tanned by the sun. Everyone has to get to know each other all over again and that is not always easy.

The newly arrived surgical team is absolutely convinced that they have to put their stamp on the hospital and the surgery department. To achieve that they totally upturn everything their predecessors have built up as soon as they arrive.

Upon the arrival of a new batch of staff it seems to be an unwritten rule for them to believe that the previous team has tackled everything incorrectly. An even bigger chaos develops.

Although the stock of sterile resources was a massive labyrinth, it was our labyrinth. We knew our way around quite well. After the arrival of the newbies we were often unpleasantly surprised when, on critical moments, we would find out that a certain item had been moved.

To be petulant I would promptly put those items, after I managed to find them, back where they used to be. This would often lead to some discontent with our new colleagues.

After doing that a few times I lose interest. I can't be bothered anymore and I rant and rave out loud when something has been moved again and I make sure I do that in both Dutch and English. I snarl that they are a bunch of morons and that they will have to find out themselves where to find everything. It is theirs from now on. I will be gone in a couple of weeks. I can't wait.

~

The number of attacks with lots of casualties increases steadily. Within a week we have to cope with two heavy hitters.

I am rudely awakened at five o'clock in the morning by the pager on the chair next to my bed. The adrenaline makes that I am immediately wide awake. On my pager's screen I read that a masscall has been announced. Upon my arrival in the hospital I get to hear there are no less than eleven casualties on the way. They are all Afghan forces who were injured during a long gun battle.

Nine of the eleven wounded were able to make it to the hospital's gate alive. The other two have received the VSA status on their way to us. They are beyond help.

After triage and stabilisation we perform surgery on six of them. Our colleagues take care of the other three. We fix bullet wounds on automatic pilot all day long and it all seems to have become so normal.

I have been quieter and more withdrawn lately. I cross off the days. I want to go home, away from this pressure cooker. The water has risen to my lips and I am starting to drown. All those times I experienced feelings that shook me to my core, I just want to forget it. I want to get back to my family to never think about this period again. When I get home, I will hand in my resignation as soon as possible. This combination of the pressure and the injuries is something I never want to experience again. The missile attacks have frightened me to death, even though they have become more 'normal'. Hopefully not a lot more will happen that is able to get to me, because I am ready to blow.

And just when I realise that, a week begins which would prove to be the proverbial last straw.

DIRECT HIT

It is Wednesday evening, 22nd August. It is quiet at Dutch Corner, the orange-coloured coffee corner. The weekly briefing has just started. Everybody listens attentively to what is being said. I am standing at the back by the bar with Linda and some other colleagues and pour myself a coffee. I suspect this coffee has been in the pot for less than an hour. I take a sniff, and decide it smells better than last time. I will take the gamble. The first sip proves I am wrong though and disgusted I swallow the stuff. I swap it for a bottle of water.

Suddenly the quiet is rudely interrupted by a door that is thrown open heavy-handedly. A young man, dressed in sportswear and with a sweaty face, pops his head around the door. For a moment he seems surprised to see so many people but then he looks around wildly and starts to shout. "Dutch surgical team! I am looking for the Dutch surgical team. Are you here? There are six alpha-status casualties on their way to us! Five Canadians and their interpreter!"

Almost immediately people begin to chat, and as if we hadn't actually heard the man, people start nudging us. Linda and I look at each other and then hurry over to the waiting guy. We make our way through the crowd. On our way out, some people wish us luck. It is obvious that by now many know what our daily job is. From all corners people call out statements of support and make sure there is room for us to get outside as quickly as possible.

In the car we hear how the pagers aren't working and that all required personnel now needs to be searched out. Once again a Canadian vehicle has driven over a mine. There are seven casualties, including a journalist and an interpreter.

"It's bad, it's very bad," the young man explains while he keeps his eyes firmly on the road.

As soon as I enter the hospital I smell an immediately familiar scent: gunpowder, diesel, blood and burnt flesh. It triggers feelings of nausea and sadness. We have no time to look at the whiteboard to see what is expected from us. From seemingly nowhere the first patient arrives in theatre. It is the interpreter who was with the Canadian unit. He looks more dead than alive. At the foot end of the operating table is the final left shoe this man has ever put on. The foot is still in it. Where his leg used to be, is now a crushed mixture of ripped uniform, flesh, dirt and dust. It is a surreal image. The pale guy lies on the operating table with a leg that hasn't got any blood running through it and that is torn to pieces. The operating room smells disgusting. It is the scent of death.

Everyone works to save his life. There is no time whatsoever to prepare the patient so he remains uncovered on the table. From all sides people shout for tools and resources. Linda and I are running to and fro to gather them all up.

No one has time to get changed into sterile clothes and no one is wearing sterile gloves either. We are already cutting into the patient.

The sound of a saw penetrates the room and within moments the patient's chest is open. The surgeons and anaesthetist are doing all they can to save this patient's life. The interpreter's heart and lungs are manually squeezed in order to keep circulation and ventilation going. It is not looking good.

The wounds don't bleed. Worse still, the only fluid that is coming from the wounds is the clear fluid we have just administered by intravenous drip. He has completely bled out.

After 20 minutes of hard work we hear that this young interpreter has become an angel. Some of those present shout swear words that seem to come from deep inside them as they storm out of the operating room. They are on their way to take care of the other casualties.

I have just put on a pair of non-sterile gloves and I am standing at the operating table. I help to suture up the deceased man's chest as neatly as possible.

I feel fat tears rolling down my cheeks, as I make stitch after stitch. Once I have finished the last stitch I clean the patient and make sure he looks as tidy as possible. With every action I take I am moved more. Once I have bandaged up the surgical wound, I look at the interpreter's face for just that bit too long. It hits me like a sledgehammer. Here on the table lies a young man. He hasn't got a beard, unlike nearly every other Afghan man I have seen. His young face is unblemished. I guess he is about my age.

I can't help but draw more parallels and by doing that I commit a capital sin: I identify with the patient. The longer I look at him, the more I become aware of my suppressed tensions that have been building up recently. Deep within me the water is churning, and it can't be constrained any longer.

We lift the deceased from the operating table to a stretcher. Just before we pull the sheet over his face, I stop at the head end for a moment. I put my hand on his left cheek. I feel the final remnants of my strength leave my body.

"I am sorry. I am so sorry."

I walk over to Linda. She is also crying and I grab her. I don't just cry for this patient. As Linda and I cling on to each other for a short while, I cry about everything, all the hidden feelings come out at this moment and she does the same. Then we grab a mop and silently clean up the operating room.

The overall sad conclusion of this evening is that two Canadian soldiers and their interpreter have lost their lives. The others all suffered minor injuries, which we took care of immediately after the interpreter. They will be flown out of Afghanistan for further treatment tomorrow.

It is around half past nine in the evening when we arrive back at Dutch Corner. The crowd of people has disappeared. Small groups of men and women are chatting together at the picnic tables behind Dutch Corner. As we sit down at an empty table, I feel all eyes on us and I hear soft mumbling.

The sports instructor, who we chat to regularly, puts some drinks in front of us. He sees our subdued looks and knows that we have had a hard time. He doesn't say a word.

Just when he wants to sit down, there is a huge blast. The ground shakes. It is almost immediately followed by another two strikes, after which the air raid sirens start to wail.

"Damn it, fucking assholes!"

I grab my drink and walk slowly to the bunker around the corner. I don't feel like running anymore as it is pointless. What are the odds the next one will hit me? In the bunker I lower myself down against the wall and light a cigarette. Deep in thought I wait till we get the all clear sign. But it wasn't the missiles that hit me. It was the interpreter.

THE WEAKEST LINK

Something in me has changed. At first it happens slowly and undetected, but this week I have started to notice it in myself. Everything I stand for - my ideals, my worldview and my self-image - has been severely affected. Where I had set myself up for just another two weeks of joining in on automatic pilot, it actually turns out to become a period during which I am moved to the core again.

The day before all of this we perform surgery on an Afghan police officer's face. It is the longest procedure of my entire deployment. I assist the surgeon for no less than fourteen continuous hours.

A flying fragment has nearly completely torn off this patient's right cheek. All the skin and muscle layers that lay in a triangle from the corner of the mouth, to behind the ear and over the nose have more or less been ripped off. This flap can be folded over the nose which makes it look like there is only half a face.

At the end of the procedure I take a deep bow at the maxillofacial surgeon. The patient has been patched up after fourteen tiring hours, which were only interrupted to quickly stretch our legs or to have a quick drink or a bite to eat. Besides the restoration of functionality, the cosmetic result is astonishing. Although I am physically broken after this day, the procedure has given me an extremely good feeling.

That is unfortunately short-lived as it disappears when I walk through the camp at the end of the day and see the Dutch flag flying at half-mast. Another colleague from our country has died as he was performing his duty. This 30-year-old sergeant perished near Deh Rawod as he tried to defuse an explosive.

The next morning a pale-faced nine-year-old boy is on the operating table. His brown eyes are calm and bright. There is no fear there, but he carefully watches everything that is going on around him. His nose has a shard wound, which we will have to reconstruct. After a three-hour long procedure, the child has a nose like before, brand new.

As we are tidying up the operating room we receive the news that our replacements are on their way. They will arrive in a couple of days, so we can begin with the HOTO, *hand-over, take-over*, the transfer. The end is near. I can finally start counting down.

In the afternoon we operate some previously admitted patients. When the last patient of the day has been helped I decide to have a look at the little patient we saw this morning. Perhaps I will give him a wave. I am known as the joker here, so the role of hospital entertainer would probably fit me well.

He is in bed under a colourful Spiderman blanket and is awake. As I walk over to him, he looks at me. He starts to cry uncontrollably when I smile at him. It shocks and upsets me. I want to help this child and say something to comfort him, but it feels like I have been rejected. I have to deal with another massive blow that shakes me to the core.

I simply stand there for a moment and then I run out of the room. Linda sees it and watches me go. The impact of what this rejection does to me eludes her. "Oh Erik, surely your kids sometimes cry too when they don't get what they want?" I hear her say as I run out of the ward. An uncontrollable rage is rising up in me.

I hide in the bunker behind the hospital. The chairs in there bear the brunt of it. I kick them over and throw them around the bunker with all my strength. There is a huge crash when they hit the concrete wall. I want to break something, but as the bunker's walls are built to withstand an incoming missile, they are able to put up with the violence of a frenzied OR nurse. With every futile attempt to tear down the bunker my frustration builds even more. I am such a failure.

Then I feel two arms around me. Linda holds me tight and feel my tears coming. I cry like a baby. I feel the ground give way and cling on to her. The discarded chairs are put back in their places. We sit down and I pour my heart out. Finally, I tell her that I am completely done. I have reached boiling point in this pressure cooker. All experiences up to now, the build-up of pressure, the severity of the injuries, the pointlessness I feel, realising that our help is not the be all and end all, the terror during the attacks and the lack of rest are finally too much.

On top of that I strongly feel that I have failed. I haven't been able to keep it together. Instead I tripped and fell. I have disappointed my colleagues. Despite the fact that I function outstandingly at the operating table, I still feel like a useless part of the team. The so-called weakest link. And that feeling of being useless lingers.

DEALING WITH THE MEDIA

I meet up with Yuri, a journalist. Blonde guy, friendly, a bit headstrong and the only person I know who smokes even more than me.

He is on his way through to Deh Rawod and will only be staying in Kandahar for a few of days. I see him a couple of times in camp where we drink a cup of coffee and smoke countless cigarettes.

Somewhere halfway through a cigarette I mention that I work in the OR and that we are swamped with work. He reacts in the same, somewhat surprised, way as many others do.

The next time we chat, he asks if I would be interested in talking about the work I do here. Perhaps he can use it for a book he plans to write. I agree.

A couple of days later I talk to him for hours about the work in theatre and the many victims we treat. I show him some pictures and videos of our daily activities. He tells me he is moved after seeing the images. I invite him to join us for a day, so he can experience up close what war surgery is about.

"You can't get any closer than that, Yuri," I say.

He immediately points out he won't be doing that. He tells me he has been through a lot lately, and that the images he has just seen have possibly woken a fear in him that he hadn't considered before. Something in him is stirring.

THE LAST MILE

My final days in Kandahar are dominated by handing over our duties to our successors. The relief team has arrived and it is good to see them again. The OR nurses who are taking over from us both have a wealth of experience. They know the ropes.

"Hand over and training are great, but we want to start working independently as quickly as possible," one of them tells us.

It is a diplomatic way of saying that they don't need our help anymore. He has only just uttered those words when I look at them gratefully and wish them all the best. They too would be heading for a hectic deployment.

I lock myself in my room. It is the only place I feel fairly okay. I hardly go outside anymore, only to smoke and to walk to the dining hall. Actually, I often skip meals. I only mingle with others once in a while. I isolate myself during those last three days.

On the penultimate day we receive a medal with a certificate from the Canadian commander of the Role 3 hospital. I just go with the flow and want to go back to my room as quickly as possible. I am completely done with it all. I have only one thing left to do here.

Lots of people have taken pictures of me because of my yellow wooden shoes. I will be leaving them behind. I ritually remove all blood splatters and tissue fragments and after a bit of polishing they look as new.

I have them screwed onto a wooden panel which includes brass plates with our names. A true memorial of our presence here. Without any embellishment I hand it over to the commander of the hospital.

DEPARTURE

It is a done deal. We are going home tomorrow. We will be flying with a Canadian C-130 Hercules tactical transport plane to the Al Minhad airbase in the United Arab Emirates. We will then travel to Dubai Airport by car and from there we will take a direct flight to Amsterdam.

On my last day in Kandahar I take pictures everywhere on the base, so I can show more than just blown up people when I get home. I have another walk around the runway and I gag one last time when I walk past Area Fifty-Poo. That is something I definitely won't miss.

I meet up with some people I saw a lot during my deployment and wish each and everyone of them the best of luck.

That last evening and night I feel restless and I wait until the last moment to pack my bags. When everyone is getting ready to go to the dining hall for breakfast I am still in my bedroom sorting out all my gear.

I am not going over to the hospital anymore because I don't feel like saying goodbye. Instead I wait till we are told we can climb the airplane's stairs.

The plane is packed. Together with at least 80 Canadian soldiers we are squashed like sardines in the cargo area. Almost everyone is sleeping with their head on the shoulder of the person next to them. I wonder what these people have been through lately.

I breathe a sigh of relief when, after flying for one and a half hours, we are told that we have left Afghan airspace. I am on my way home! When we arrive at Al Minhad in the UAE we receive the warmest of welcomes with a delicious meal and cold soft drinks. We are allocated a container, where we can shower and change into civilian clothes. Because we depart from the civilian airport in Dubai we have to travel in civilian clothes. It makes me smile. Are we not allowed to stand out? Five people in jeans with combat boots carrying heavy camouflage duffel bags, will definitely not stand out from the crowds, I think sarcastically.

A few hours later we get on the big blue KLM plane that will fly us directly to Amsterdam where my wife and parents will be waiting for me.

We are not going to Crete to adapt. We are not given any time to get used to the fact that we are no longer living with war, we aren't given time for the adrenaline levels to drop. Mine are still very high. I look over my shoulder a lot and I am hyper alert.

Immediately after landing in Amsterdam we change back into our desert-coloured uniforms. Although we are at the back of a long queue of people, we are quickly noticed by our colleagues from the military police. "Welcome home, job well done," the blonde guy says as he waves us through.

An emotional reunion with my wife and parents follows. The commander of the hospital I work is waiting for us too. Well-meant, but I hardly notice him. I don't feel any need for it and I want to go home straight away, to be with my family. I say goodbye to my colleagues. I am back home!

It seems strange to me that everyone is walking around the airport without a care in the world. Some are wearing flip flops, shorts and t-shirts. These people aren't worried about anything, whilst at the same time a war is raging in my head. My thoughts are running away from me.

Where is my pager? I forgot to put my pager in my pocket! It is so busy here. The perfect spot to cause a lot of damage. Then I realise I am in the Netherlands. I have left the war, but only physically. I don't want to think about the period behind me anymore. Everything that happened, was back in Kandahar and I want to leave it there. I want to go home as quickly as possible to see my boys.

BUSINESS AS USUAL

"Daddy!" Mika and Lars jump up simultaneously when I walk into the room. They hang off my leg and it looks like they won't ever let go again. I hug them for a long time, sit them on my lap and hold them close, whispering sweet words and kissing both of them.

The house and garden are decorated with bunting. It is an amazing day. I tell everybody I am ecstatic to be home again, but don't tell them about my experiences. All I say is that it was busy. And hot, boiling hot. I don't want to talk about it anymore, as they won't get it anyway. No one will ever be able to understand or feel what I have seen, felt and experienced there. For that you have to have been there.

That same afternoon I walk to the supermarket. I push the trolley around in a daze and watch all the people around me. Again, I think about how strange it feels for me to be walking around here while my colleagues are fighting for their lives over there.

I see a lady complaining to an employee of the supermarket that a certain coffee is out of stock. I stop to look at the scene. I cannot understand why she is so upset, she is going ballistic.

"Act normal! It is only coffee," I mumble as I nod my head, sigh, and walk away.

"Stupid people. You're all spoiled here!"

Visitors come and go and I see lots of people who are all happy that I am back. During their visits I am not really present though. They all have the same burning question, about how it was, but I avoid answering it. Slowly but surely I am getting more tense.

Three days after I get back home I walk into town with my wife. As I am trying on new shoes, the shop owner asks me where I got my tan. Indifferently I tell him that I have just arrived back home from Afghanistan.

"What did you do there?" he asks.

I tell him that I worked over there as an OR nurse and that it has been very busy.

"Ah well, blood has the same colour wherever you are. It's nothing special, is it," he says without looking up.

As he walks off to get some shoes for me in another size I feel the blood draining from my face. I shake with anger and clench my fists. All my senses are sharpened, I am ready to attack and want to follow him to punch his lights out.

"Nothing special? Fuck you, you fucking moron!" I whisper.

My wife notices what is happening, hears me swear and grabs my arm. She pushes me out of the shop with gentle force. I have never been back to that shop.

DOWNHILL

When I return to the surgery department of the hospital where I work after my leave, I don't seem to be able to find my feet. I no longer enjoy surgery nor do I enjoy the contact with people and I reluctantly go to work. The only one I want to talk to is Linda as I distance myself as much as possible from everyone and everything. I only do what is expected from me in my job, and absolutely nothing else. I also don't talk about how I feel. I carry on like that for a couple of weeks and I know what I need to do.

I have requested a meeting with the commander of the hospital, to let him know about my plan to resign and to ask for his permission. I don't want this job anymore, never again do I want to end up in a hell like the one I have just returned from. As I don't want to go on another deployment I strongly feel that I should leave the army on the first possible occasion. Deployments are an important part of the deal as military personnel and I feel that there is no longer a place for people in the armed forces if they don't want to be deployed anymore.

A few months after I get home I go downhill. It feels like a tiger has awakened in me and it is waiting to strike. I start to walk away from home. First it is just innocent walking, but it results in leaving the house almost compulsively. Without saying a word, I walk out of the door more often and stay away longer too.

I get an ominous feeling most evenings and I hear sounds that aren't actually there. I recognise them from Kandahar. I don't sleep well and am often troubled by memories. I cut myself off from my wife and children at home and don't utter a word about Afghanistan. My evenings are spent in front of my laptop just so that I don't have to answer any questions from my home front. I stick with this strategy of avoidance and refine it to perfection. I become a true professional in diverting difficult conversations and dodging tricky questions.

I show people what they expect from me and what they want to see. With surgical precision I cut everything and everyone that gets too close to my core out of my life. I want to pretend that the entire deployment never happened, that my memories aren't real as I consciously choose to bury my head in the sand.

ESCAPING

"Where are you? Are you coming home?"

I can hear the tension in my wife's voice as soon as I answer the phone. It is tipping down and I am soaked. The biting wind numbs my face, as I look around in a daze and realise I have no idea where I am. Only when I retrace my steps I actually recognise the surroundings and I see that I am miles away from home.

"I'm on my way, baby. Why don't you go to bed?"

I curse as I put my phone in my pocket and speed up. I walk along a long, straight country road. In some places there is a lamppost. In the dim light of one of them I try to look at my watch. I have to wipe the raindrops off the face of it before I can see what time it is. It is nearly midnight. I have been gone for an hour and a half.

Before I walked out of the door I was sitting at the kitchen table. The coffee my wife had poured for me had gone cold. I had hardly spoken a word that evening, as my thoughts kept wandering off to what I had seen, done and experienced these past few months in Afghanistan. I simply sat there staring into space, my eyes glazed over.

One by one the memories came flooding back and slowly I got sucked into all that happened over there. These were impressions I was desperate to forget, but the harder I tried, the faster they came back. All I wanted was to clear my head. Without a word I walked out of the door, leaving my wife behind, alone and confused.

I walk back with big steps and grumble at myself, the weather, the whole world. How did I end up here and what did I pass on the way? Where was my head at? Probably at Kandahar, southern Afghanistan. At least it was warm over there, I think sarcastically.

I pull up my collar and put my hands in my pockets. A car speeds past behind me. It makes me jump and I step in a puddle. I groan and look down at my feet. I expect to see water splashing up my trainers. I look again because where I thought I would see my 'civvy shoes' they seem to have been replaced by desert boots. Instead of water splashing up from the puddle, I stir up fine sand and dust with every step I take. Lightning and the subsequent thunder put me on edge. Suddenly I realise where I am.

Somewhat ashamed I walk into our house. My wife is sitting on the sofa and I notice she looks at me from head to toe. I see fear in her eyes as she starts to talk. "I've been terrified, Erik. You were gone for such a long time. And then it started to rain the way it did. Where have you been?"

I take off my coat and put it on a chair to dry out. "I walked the long way around and only realised I'd have to walk all the way back when it started to rain," I lie with a smile. "Nothing's going to happen to me, darling. I'm not stupid. Though you probably wouldn't agree seeing the state I arrived home in," I try, jokingly.

She can't laugh about it. She has been worried sick.

The next day my mum tells me off after she finds out I was away for such a long time. "You scared your wife to death. Don't ever do that again!" She looks worried.

Everyone seems to worry about me, but I let them get on with it. Stoically I sit down at the kitchen table, switch on my computer and stare at my screen. I don't explain what is up with me, because not saying a thing is what I am good at.

FIRST TREATMENT

A few weeks after my deployment I come in contact with Yuri again. He has just returned from another trip to Afghanistan and he tells me that shortly after he returned home he flipped during a visit to the pub and that he 'used his fists'. A flash of recognition as I have also had the feeling that I was ready to explode.

My spring is still in its box, but the lock that keeps the lid in place is getting weaker. That time I was in town with Harriette to buy shoes and the salesman made that inappropriate comment almost made the lid pop off the box.

We talk about our long conversation in Kandahar during which he pointed out he didn't want to see too much of the work we did in the hospital. Something awoke in him after our chat that probably had been slumbering for quite a while and it sometimes bothers him. I tell him that I have been really troubled by some memories lately, talk about my sleepless nights and concentration problems and that I have also experienced some flashbacks. We wish each other luck and make sure we know that we are here for each other if need be.

The last thing that I tell him is that it 'might be some sort of PTSD', but that I will be able to handle it, because, just like I have said so many times before: PTSD only happens to others!

"I don't know what's up with me, but I'll make sure it goes away, as quickly as possible," I write to him. I really try to make these words a reality, but I simply can't forget some images and it makes me anxious. The only way I find peace and quiet is by walking. I walk to empty my head and as the weeks go on I walk more often and for longer periods of time.

My wife is worried to death and is angry with me as I try and laugh away her concerns. Behind my contrived laugh is a much deeper problem. One I am aware of and that won't leave of its own accord. The first dents in my armour have started to appear.

My family confronts me about me walking away and about the fact my wife is worried, but I try to be the joker for them too. I promise both Harriette and my family that I will inform the Defence Department that there are things I want to talk about.

I soon get that opportunity, because a follow-up day has been planned by the unit that deployed me. It will be the first reunion of the team I was a member of during those weeks in the desert.

Lots has happened since the deployment and everyone is dealing with it in their own way. However, we don't sit down together to talk about our experiences. We simply receive our medals and have a one-to-one with someone from the social services team within the Ministry of Defence. I tell her that I am struggling with only a couple of things and that my family has noticed that too.

I make a huge mistake by not sharing more details and by not talking more freely. I mention that I would like to talk about some patients we treated in Afghanistan who now visit me in my sleep. Immediately I decide though that I will bury my head in the sand again as soon as I get rid of those nightly visitors. I will keep going as if nothing has ever happened.

167

After this chat I get the assurance that I can arrange an appointment with Military Mental Healthcare Department in a city near my hometown, where I will start a counselling programme.

Not long after, the difficult and intense talks about some of the things I experienced start. I carefully choose what experiences I want to share.

In hindsight I make a mistake again by not being more open. Instead of talking about all I have been through openly and transparently, I choose some occasions I can and want to talk about. The rest remains untouched in my head. I want to let it all rest there, to never touch it again.

According to my practitioner, these few handpicked, traumatic experiences would be very suitable for EMDR therapy: *Eye Movement Desensitisation and Reprocessing.*

I am transferred to Jeff, a psychologist who is qualified to provide EMDR therapy. I would be in touch with him much more than I could have suspected.

EMDR is a treatment that is used for people who have PTSD, or who have been through other traumatic experiences. It is mostly used to help people work through these experiences.

At the beginning of such a session we pick a specific experience. I need to think back and focus on the most painful part of that event. Focusing on that often gives me an unpleasant feeling somewhere in my body. I then tell the psychologist where that feeling is, and what negative thought comes up. Then I have to explain which positive thought I would prefer to feel with that image instead. Finally, he asks me how bad it is on a scale from one to ten to look at this image.

I have to wear headphones and think of the image, whilst I randomly hear clicks in either my left or right ear for one minute. After that minute the clicks stop and I have to name the first thing that comes to mind. Then I have to focus on that thought and a new series of clicks follows. This is repeated a couple of times, so that I can name all associations I have with that original image.

After doing this a few times I am asked to think back to the original image. There is often a noticeable change in my experience already. For example, where the score was a definite ten before, after a session this could well be a nine or eight. Repetition follows until the score is sufficiently low to be able to look calmly at this traumatic image. It often takes multiple sessions to get to such a low score.

As soon as the load of the original memory is decreased, I express the positive thought I would like to see connected to the image, and give this new truth a number on the scale from one to seven. I then focus on that statement and another series of clicks follows. This is repeated until the score is increased to a six or sometimes even a seven. This can also take a lot of sessions.

Finally the therapist asks if I feel any physical tension with the image, anywhere in my body. It took a lot of sessions before I was able to look calmly at some of the images connected to multiple experiences, but it does help. It is like a professional sport and I am absolutely wrecked when I come out of the room. I need a day, most of the time several days to recover from it. Thoughts and feelings are slung to and fro, but it is worth it.

The way EMDR works isn't completely clear yet. A possible explanation could be that remembering a traumatic event in combination with focusing on the clicks through the headphones (some therapists also use a finger the patient needs to follow) make that the natural processing system is activated. The patient uses a lot of memory capacity when a traumatic event is remembered, as this memory is vivid and very intense. Following the sounds and/or the therapist's finger during EMDR therapy also uses the working memory capacity. There seems to be some sort of a competition between the working memory tasks and because of this there is less room for the vividness and intensity of the memory. As a result, the patient will eventually be able to give another meaning to the traumatic memory.

~

After some weeks of therapy I receive good news from the armed forces. My resignation request has been approved. After fourteen years of loyal service I will leave my role with the army in May, to start my new job the very next day. My ex-colleague and, by now, good friend Marc has offered me a job and it is completely different from my current work, with a chance of normal civilian life.

I want to cut all ties with the armed forces as soon as I am back in civil life, including the talks and therapy with Military Mental Health Department. I soon try and tell myself and the psychologist that I can do it all on my own again. Although my practitioner openly doubts this, I shake his hand two months later.

"Don't take it personally, Jeff, but I hope to never see you again," I say with a smile when I leave.

As soon as I say my final goodbye to Defence, I have a period during which I feel quite good. I have a new challenge and because of that there is no reason to look back at the past year. However, I still sometimes wake up in the middle of the night because something has scared me, or because I feel like something terrible is about to happen.

KEEP GOING

My new job is the best distraction I could have wished for, because I can focus on it every minute of the day. The more I work, the less I worry and because of this I work harder and longer. I often work during weekends too and I keep going in an unhealthy way. My days are too long and I don't rest enough, but I know that every minute I spend on focusing on business, I can not think about Afghanistan.

Even on my days off and during holidays I make sure that I always have my phone with me, or that my laptop is within easy reach. My job is my ultimate escape. On days that I feel good, I work hard because I feel positive, and on the days I don't, I work even harder so I don't have time to worry.

I slowly change from the carefree guy I thought I was into the sort of pathological workaholic I never wanted to be. I notice I am less accessible to the people around me and my family suffers because of it. When I sit and work at the table and my boys come over to play a game with me, I sometimes tell them no and send them away. Seeing the disappointment in their eyes doesn't make me feel good, but it does happen.

"You're always working. Don't forget about your family and friends," they complain. They are right, but I can't help it. I have to work, as that is how I manage to suppress most of my memories. My head is so full of other thoughts that there is not a lot of room for painful things.

I sometimes feel bad. When I look in the mirror in the morning I see a reasonably successful man who does everything he can for the business, but at the expense of himself and the ones who are dear to him.

My world is slowly getting smaller. Brick by brick I build a wall around myself, which is able to withstand all external influences, but also the forces from within. Even the strongest wall can get damaged though, its bricks can eventually loosen and its integrity will then be undermined. I know it, I see what is happening, but I don't do anything about it. I just keep going.

Three years after coming home I get back in touch with Yuri. I am in front of my computer cleaning up some files. I am just about to delete the email address I used in Afghanistan when I notice an invite for Yuri's book launch in that mailbox. The date for the event was a week ago, so I decide to contact him directly. I apologise and tell him I would have loved to attend.

He tells me that he has included the conversation we had in Kandahar in his book. That August night in the Afghan desert was powerful for him and it was the same for me. A couple of weeks later we meet up and talk for a long time about that dreadful summer.

I tell him I have left the armed forces. It feels good to talk to Yuri, as I have a feeling that he actually understands. He has been there and he knows.

"Do you still work in the operating room, or are you completely done with that?"

I tell him that I am as good as done with it and that I am very happy in my new job.

~

Once in a while I still work as an OR nurse in a clinic near my hometown through my new employer's company.

There I get to work with a really nice team and I meet Sebastian, a plastic surgeon who I immediately get on with. We have the same absurd sense of humour, and we both share the same passion: music. I really enjoy working with him. We get talking during surgery and he sometimes asks me about the work of an OR nurse within the armed forces. When he asks if I have been deployed lately, I tell him that I was in a huge sandbox not that long ago. And that it was warm and busy, but also that I saw and did horrendous things over there, without going into details. He can picture what I am talking about as a surgical specialist.

A couple of weeks later we are in the clinic's coffee room together. Suddenly the whining sound of the fire alarm sounds through the whole building. I drop myself down on my stomach in a reflex. It takes a couple of seconds before I realise that there won't be a missile.

"Are you looking for something?"

When I look up, I see Sebastian standing over me with a big grin on his face.

I quickly get up and start laughing too.

"Afghanistan?" he asks.

It is a question I can only answer with a yes.

Sebastian would become my best friend.

LETTING IT ALL OUT

The first confrontation with myself happens five years after my deployment.

Before that time I did everything in my power to block all memories and that is how I kept it all together. There were lots of moments when some things surfaced, but I just pretended they weren't there and kept on going; specifically on the annually recurring dates when something had happened during my deployment in Afghanistan that really affected me, or when something shown on television suddenly sparked a memory.

I pushed it away and threw myself into my work, but I felt Afghanistan was catching up with me. I looked over my shoulder and saw it coming. I would erect all my walls one last time and it was at this exact moment that one of my best friends died.

~

I had known him for many years. He was a true eccentric. He was always up for a chat and I visited him often. In fact, he was the last person I visited, before I left to the airport on the day that I flew to

Afghanistan. Though he had lost his job, he never complained and he never asked for help. Gradually he drank more and more, and eventually he didn't take care of himself or his household anymore. I worried about him, but he didn't allow anyone to guide or help him, as he was simply too proud.

Over the years he changed from an energetic man into a drinker who would only sit on the sofa. I would visit him a couple of times a week, to help him tidy up his house and also for social control. I always took into account that I would find him dead on his sofa one day, with a half-full glass and an extinguished cigarette between his fingers.

Around Christmas that year he dies from the complications of an acute gastric bleed. When I hear this, I fall apart. I hadn't seen him for a couple of days and had knocked on his door several times. It was in vain. My fear has become reality.

The days leading up to the cremation I feel bad and I notice I can't help thinking about it at night. I think about all the fun times we had, but also about how lonely he must have felt and how he, certainly during his last days, must have felt so poorly. Eventually he vomited blood and crawled to the shower to die there. I try and block that from my mind, like I often do with images that touch my soul.

After the cremation I continue to feel upset for days. It seems harder to distance myself from it all, also because my boys still regularly ask questions about him. During those moments I feel the sharp pains of loss. He didn't want to be helped and I couldn't help him.

From time to time in the depth of the night I suddenly see the whiteboard that used to hang on the wall at the Role 3 hospital, displaying the announcement about six Canadian soldiers who were on their way to our hospital. I see how the writing on the whiteboard is erased. I think about these Canadians we couldn't save and about my dear friend whom I couldn't save. I draw parallels of self-accusation.

I don't take any time out for myself, because I know there is more going on than simply grieving my friend. Something is stirring deep within me and I sometimes feel the dry desert heat, and I often smell a sickly scent that makes me heave. I know what it is, but I never want to get close to those memories ever again. For now, I am still standing, but I feel I am faltering.

I experience another big blow later that year. A close acquaintance ends her life and I am shocked. It awakens the memory of losing a very dear friend through suicide years ago. For the time being I somehow manage to suppress that painful memory. It is getting harder though and the cracks in my wall get deeper and deeper as the chance of it crumbling to pieces is becoming a reality.

The summer holidays are good, except for the dates that come back to bite me yearly, because on those days something major happened in Kandahar. Straight after the holidays I fall back into my old habit of working obsessively so that I don't have time to think about other things. That autumn I start to develop physical complaints and it all goes wrong at the end of the year during a business trip in Germany.

I fall ill at the hotel where I am staying. My temperature is very high, I have an excruciating stomach ache and can't stop being sick. The colic cramps paired with excessive spasms make that I cannot lie still and the pain is driving me insane. I think I am developing a gastric bleed, just like my dear friend. I can't shake the image of me being all alone in my hotel room, crawling to the shower to die.

That night I am scared and ill and as a result I hardly sleep. The next morning my business contact takes me to the local hospital. After some examinations it appears that I have an acutely infected gallbladder that needs immediate surgery. I insist that I will be treated in a hospital in near home, so the colleague who joined me on this trip takes me back home.

I admit myself to the hospital where I worked at the surgery department for three years. In the OR it is an absurd reunion with my colleagues. Everyone greets me warmly.

"I've missed you guys and I do anything I can to see you again," I joke. Then my face contorts in pain. When it is time for anaesthetics, something flashes before my eyes: suddenly I am no longer in this operating room, but in the Role 3 hospital in Kandahar. It makes me jump. The image disappears as quickly as it appears.

"Don't pay any attention to me talking gibberish about what I saw and did in Afghanistan, when I am falling asleep. Don't pay any attention to me when I am unsettled whilst waking up or when I tell you stupid things. I am scared, so fucking scared of the memories!" Panic washes over me.

I feel the hand of the nurse anaesthetist on my shoulder. An ex-colleague is standing next to me and places her hand on my lower arm and then I hear exactly the same words I said numerous of times in Afghanistan. "We're going to take real good care of you, Erik. Find yourself a nice dream and inhale deeply. Don't worry about anything. Sleep tight."

I stay in hospital for a couple of days after my surgery. I don't sleep well and notice the sleeping tiger in me is waking up.

SOMETHING ON MY MIND

It is getting increasingly difficult for me to find the energy for the things I need to do. This feeling has been growing ever since my gallbladder was removed some months ago.

I feel really tense and I am irritable when I am at home. I keep snapping at people. Even though I am aware of it, I don't do anything to stop it. I regularly have bad headaches and heart palpitations. People warn me that I am at risk of developing a burnout. After all, I am always working.

To make sure I look after myself a bit better, I start to exercise fanatically. This would prove to be an important outlet for me later that year. I am no longer able to use my work as a way of escaping. I have reached the limit and I can't work any harder. My head feels full, it is getting too much.

Repeatedly I see all sorts of images; a flash of a patient without an arm or without legs on the operating table or a body that is shot to pieces. I am able to tell myself that it is an illusion. Only just though.

A couple of months after the surgery my body pulls the emergency cord once again. I develop the same stomach cramps as I had before the gallbladder operation, and end up in hospital again. Blood tests show that my liver values are way too high. They immediately do an X-ray of my upper abdomen. In the distance I hear the gentle ringing of alarm bells. The echo shows a shadow, a spot on my liver. I am told this could simply be some scar tissue from the previous gallbladder operation, but it could also be a tumour. The alarm bells that were ringing softly in the distance now swell to a deafening noise. It really frightens me and my thoughts run away with me. I feel like I have won the 'top prize' and I should go and choose a coffin right now.

I will be transferred to another hospital for additional examinations. On my way there I put on a brave face and tell myself that I should not be worried, as it is probably only scar tissue. But once in the hospital I get more scared with every step I take.

I break down during my admission talk with the nurse and I cry because of my fear of death. I remember that I felt like this before; when the missiles hit base. I am just as scared here in this hospital as I was then in the bunker!

I am examined again the next day, but there is still no decisive answer and because of this I have to stay another few days.

In the middle of the night I get the fright of my life. There is a massive blow in the corridor. I feel the rush of adrenaline through my body and before I know it I am face down on the floor next to my bed, shaking like a leaf. My left hand hurts. It is because the IV drip got ripped out when I took a nosedive to the ground. Blood is dripping from where the needle was just a moment ago. I ring for the nurse and tell her that I wasn't feeling well and stepped out of the bed on the wrong side without thinking straight. "I was probably half-asleep, and completely forgot about the needle in my hand," I stammer.

She gives me a new drip and stares at me for a while, as if she is waiting for me to tell her what really happened.

"Sleep tight, Erik, do ring us if there is anything you need," she says, smiling warmly.

I smile at her too, sheepishly. I feel the same fear as during my deployment when we were shot at with rockets. Earlier today I was scared to death, and now I feel like that again, because of that blow. I realise something is definitely wrong with me.

The ball that has been carefully pushed under water is about to come up with brute force. I am scared of it, scared to lose control and to be flooded with negative memories.

I phone Sebastian from my hospital bed. "It happened again, dude. I was on the floor again."

It is quiet on the other end of the phone.

I tell him about the blast I heard at night and that I was suddenly lying next to my bed.

He doesn't laugh this time.

I have some more examinations in hospital, but none of them seem to be able to give an explanation for my symptoms, my blood counts and the shadow on my liver. I have turned completely yellow over the last couple of days. Then my temperature suddenly drops and my elevated liver functions also slowly return to normal levels again. My last examination is an MRI scan, showing that the shadow on my liver is actually scar tissue from the previous gallbladder operation.

A weight has been lifted off my shoulders. The reason for the elevated liver functions will never be found. It doesn't matter to me. I am going home.

Back at home, I rest for a couple of days and try to calm the ever-increasing chaos in my head, which I can't. Though I am getting better physically, mentally I am slipping. I have not really been able to sleep since my hospitalisation, and when I look in the mirror, I see a guy I hardly recognise. What a wreck, what a sad figure. I am ashamed of myself and my head is jam-packed, leaving no space to feel joy or even to focus on trivial things.

REACHING OUT

I am in a constant bad mood and often feel emotional. I also feel terribly restless. I have been told in hospital that I have high blood pressure, which doesn't come as a surprise to me. The pressure inside of me has been increasing for too long. The lid of Pandora's Box is coming off soon, I can feel it.

That moment comes a couple weeks later, during a conversation with a social worker in my company. Suddenly I break down and explain that I can no longer suppress the memories I have been burying for six years and that I am drowning. I feel like I am back in Afghanistan.

A box of tissues is pushed in front of me and after an hour of spilling my guts I walk out of the door, shaking and tense, feeling terrible and overwhelmed. I smoke a couple of cigarettes in the car, realising I shouldn't drive in this state, because I would cause an accident, intentionally or unintentionally. I can't stop crying. I utter an animalistic scream and ram my fist against the roof. I ring my wife in a panic and say that I am not doing well at all. Finally the Afghan tiger is wide awake and has caught up with me.

Sobbing, I look through the cards in my wallet. It is as if, during all those years of hiding away myself and my memories, I have always known that this particular day would come. I must have a card from the *Veterans Institute* (VI) somewhere in my wallet.

I curse myself for sinking so low. I am going crazy and I am scared to get locked up, like I am a danger to myself and the people around me. I can't take it alone anymore, I will have to ring them.

The warm voice on the other end of the line tries to reassure me. I apologise for my broken voice and explain I am in the car and that I am panicking. Every word of it is true. I answer lots of questions and am told I will be phoned back right away. Less than five minutes after I put the phone down a social worker from the armed forces rings me. I have a long and emotional conversation with her and she manages to calm me down slowly. "We're going to help you, Erik. We're here to look after you," she assures me.

An appointment is planned for the next day. That same social worker will come and do an intake with me to get a clear idea of my issues. I have to solemnly swear that after this phone call I will stay in the car till I am calmer. I will then drive home carefully and stay with my loved ones for the rest of the day.

She also tells me that it is okay to cry, to be angry and sad. I don't have to take care of myself on my own anymore, they are going to help me.

The first thing I do when I get home is hold my wife and cry.

I then tell her and the kids that I think a lot about my time in Afghanistan and that it makes me really sad. I cry even harder when the boys give me a big hug.

"You're a hero, daddy."

It is beautiful weather on the day of my intake appointment. I sit in the garden as I smoke a roll-up when the doorbell rings. It is the social worker of the organisation that does the intake on behalf of the Veterans Institute.

I pour her a cup of tea and we talk for a long time as we sit at the kitchen table. I get turned inside out.

I tell her how I have buried everything for years, but that I can't do it anymore. I am tortured by memories all day long and have flashbacks that cause fear, despondency, powerlessness and anger.

I am ashamed that I haven't managed to remain upright. Not in Afghanistan nor at home. Can it get any worse? I know I need help and I ask for it. "Please help me. Help me."

Another three conversations follow after the first one, which my wife is part of too. She jumps in where needed and explains how hard I have been working and that I have slowly become unavailable to everyone and everything. It hurts to hear what I have done to my family.

The aid worker brings her report along at the last appointment. It is about all that seems to be going on, and I am allowed to read it. Then I get asked what I think that would help me. I indicate that I would like to go back to the Military Mental Health Department. I absolutely do not want to be seen by a civilian psychologist, as I feel that someone who has never been deployed in the desert won't be able to help me.

"They wouldn't get it. If you haven't been there, you won't get it. Only the ones who have been deployed themselves will understand."

She is going to look into it and within a week an appointment has been made with a psychologist of the Military Mental Health Department.

I can go and see Jeff, the same therapist I told I hoped I would never see again when I said goodbye to him five years ago.

FIGHT OR FLIGHT

"Who would have thought it? So, we do see each other again. Welcome back!" Jeff smiles as he shakes my hand firmly. I try to smile, but I just can't.

Finally, I am going to get help. I know that I have a long way to go and that it has only just started. This time I will really have to open up and however difficult I think talking is, I will battle with myself and my ghosts. I won't walk away from it any longer. However long it will take and however hard it will get, I will completely empty this poisoned chalice.

The appointments that follow are exhausting. I feel worse every time and get the feeling that more and more rubbish is being stirred up. I am being torn down instead of being built up. Every single conversation I get asked for more details, including the ones I don't want to share.

For weeks I don't sleep more than a few hours per night. I often wake up to thoughts running through my head. I am advised to, when I wake up, immediately note down keywords about what I see, hear, think, and feel. Writing down apparently creates a calm feeling.

It only proves to be partially true. I can't seem to organise the chaos in my head and I am not really able to concentrate. When I leave the house to go and buy a loaf of bread, I find myself in the supermarket five minutes later without actually knowing what I am there for. I then ring home to ask about it, with tears in my eyes, feeling like a failure. I have gone mad and I have done that myself. It is all my fault and I feel so ashamed.

This can not be true. I didn't even leave the base in Afghanistan, where the real danger was. All I did was work at the operating room, like I did at home, but I couldn't carry on. I have let the experiences get to me and they have become too much to deal with. Yet, I am able to look at it rationally too: the number of patients, the limited capacity, the lack of rest and the intensity of the traumas have all led to it getting too much.

My head tells me that it is not that strange. Never ever have my head and my heart been that far apart.

THE PEN IS MIGHTIER THAN
THE SWORD

"Bring your guitar," Sebastian says, just before he puts down the phone.

I am going to visit him in the hope that I will be able to relax for a day. We will also be making music together. In his studio the two of us will start recording some tracks that are special to me. Most of these songs were played often in the operating room in Kandahar. I can hardly listen to them without crying.

For the first time in a very long time I have a good day. We laugh a lot, cry a lot and we have long conversations only true friends can have. I enjoy our friendship and the common passion for music and our shared goal.

At lunchtime we sit at the kitchen table and have a lengthy chat about working through trauma. Recently, Sebastian and his wife Marilyn have also experienced a very traumatic life event. He surprises me when he tells me that he has been thinking a lot about me because of that, and that he is now able to understand a bit more what trauma can do to someone.

During my sessions with Jeff we elaborate on my experiences. Since I started my treatment last year, I have told some people that I am struggling with what I experienced in Afghanistan.

"It's probably PTSD," I tell them.

I even mention to a friend at judo that I have started to wrestle with whether I should carry on or give up. I tell her I have had enough of my life.

"Erik, you might well be on your back on the floor, but you're not going to tap out! You can't tap out!"

Her words bring tears to my eyes. It would become my motto.

A couple of days later when I see Jeff I ask why I keep feeling this bad, even though I am now working so hard to get rid of the ghosts from the past. Jeff doesn't hesitate and says: "That's exactly what PTSD does to you, Erik."

Although I have suspected it for a while, this is actually the first time that a professional confirms that I have a serious problem. I am diagnosed with PTSD. It feels like recognition and it sends shivers down my spine.

It is during this conversation that Jeff asks me to find my little diary from Kandahar and write down what I did in Afghanistan day by day. This will provide more structure in my head and to my experiences. I also find it easier to write things down than to actually say them. As soon as I have described a given day I will pass it on to Jeff. He will note down further questions and comments, which we will talk through together.

TRIPPING OVER

In the attic the TL light buzzes into life. I climb the stairs with a heavy heart. Once upstairs I stop. My eyes shoot across the room. To the left is a pile of untouched moving boxes. They were put here after the move and have never been looked at again. Why didn't I just get rid of them? Angry, I decide to throw them all out very soon. If they have been here for months and nothing has been done with them, they can be thrown away.

Subconsciously I draw a parallel with what is in my head. The memories have been there for years, but nothing has been done with them. It is high time to clear them.

All the way at the back, hidden behind yet more boxes, I find what I am looking for: two heavy, army-green duffel bags. Reluctantly I open the first bag and immediately I am overwhelmed by emotions. I sit down and cry my eyes out. Sobbing, I empty all the contents on the attic floor.

A fat, closed envelope attracts my attention. I sniff once again, wipe away my tears and start opening it with shaking hands. The weighty Next of Kin Handbook appears. I had agreed with my wife to get rid

190

of it straight after my return. I haven't even been able to do that. Annoyed, I throw the heavy manual down from the top of the stairs.

After a bit more digging through the stuff I find what I was looking for; the diary that I kept during my deployment.

I grab it and look at it for a moment. I trace the hard cover with my index finger and clench the little book between my hands. Without even having to open it, all the events resurface one by one. They fill me with long forgotten emotions.

Some dates from my deployment pop into my head. I am on my knees with my eyes closed. Images fill my head. I leaf through the diary slowly. My stomach hurts and I feel nauseous. Now and then I have a sour taste in my mouth.

The first pages are filled with clear and detailed descriptions of the day. The further I read, the shorter and darker the notes become. They are no longer that elaborate and are laced with anger and disillusion. Eventually, there are even days without any notes at all. During these I was too busy to write anything. All I wanted to do after surgery on those particular days was sleep.

It is also possible I wanted to forget about that day straight away, so I consciously didn't write anything about it. I don't have to read anything about the days with empty diary pages anyway. The blank days force themselves upon me like a film constantly playing in my head. A film that cannot be stopped.

I close it as soon as I see the page with the six names of the Canadians we couldn't save. I have seen enough and feel exactly like I did the day we said our goodbyes to them.

With big steps and without looking up or down I hurtle down the attic stairs. There are only another three steps to go when I slip and, with a dull thud followed by loud curse, I end up on my back on the landing.

The back of my head hits the floor. When I get up I touch the back of my head. It is spinning. I look at my hand and expect to see blood. I don't, though it will probably become a bruise. My head is banging from the pain and I am angry with myself.

What just happened? I look around in a daze when I see the ripped open envelope and the book I just slipped over. Ironically, I could have broken my neck over the Next of Kin Handbook.

On the dinner table is the usual mess of my kids' school stuff. My laptop is on a cleared part of the table with its screen flipped up. An empty page is open in the word-processing programme. This is going to be the first page of the story I promised myself I would never tell.

I have been staring at the screen for quite some time. My fingers fly restlessly across the keyboard. Pieces of text appear on the screen and every single piece is removed as quickly as it appears. Thoughts pop in and out of my head. I am being thrown to and fro. It is too hectic in my head.

To try and organise it all, my psychologist has indicated that I have to write everything down. But where do I start?

Not talking about my memories and pushing them away has become second nature. I know I need help and I am now getting it, but I would still rather not talk at all. I am afraid of the memories, and I fear that, when I tell others about them, they will have as bad an opinion about me as I have. And that is very bad indeed.

Once we have taken stock of my problems during a string of lengthy sessions, it is decided that I am going to receive EMDR treatment for the most painful memories, just like I did some years ago.

All these sessions, every single one as gruelling as the next one, should help me to be able to view the images I have been so afraid of in a calmer way.

Till the end of that year I try and sort out my head, but I don't notice any improvement, as I am still not able to concentrate or sleep properly and I am constantly on edge. I want to run away from it all again, like I did years ago.

I get that chance when Jeff tells me a couple weeks later that he is due to be deployed for four months.

He asks if I would be okay with him temporarily handing me over to one of his colleagues. I tell him I don't want that and I say that I am more than capable to handle those few weeks without him and that we can pick up where we left off as soon as he gets back.

I know that that is nowhere near the truth, but I see it as an opportunity to be free from difficult conversations for a couple of weeks. We continue with the tough sessions and the EMDR until he leaves in April.

In the weeks he is gone I go downhill rapidly. My head is close to exploding. I do anything I can to function the way that is expected from me, but in everything I do I notice that I am deteriorating.

Even memories that I have never spoken about before come to the surface and make me feel bad. I can't escape the feeling that I am failing. I feel powerless, I have done it all wrong. Both during my deployment, when I allowed myself to be torn down, and in the period after it, when I pretended that I was able to manage it all.

I don't sleep a lot at night, which makes me more vulnerable during the day, which in turn means there are more images at night and that makes me sleep even less. It is a vicious circle I can't escape from.

Gradually, I become more and more depressed and can't enjoy fun things anymore. I hardly notice any progress. I know that I can't expect something that has been building for six years to be sorted in less than a year, but even with the help I now receive I am not getting any better.

The memories are slowly falling into their places though. The casuistry, the patients, start to lose their connotation, but the overall feeling about the deployment and about myself is causing issues. Lots of veterans are proud of their status, but I am experiencing the exact opposite. I feel outright terrible that I have been over there and it feels like I am still in the middle of it all. I am a shadow of the man I thought I was.

Not long ago I had to admit reluctantly that I couldn't handle dealing with my memories on my own. I am so disappointed and I am so extremely angry at myself. In the mirror I see a man with red circles under his eyes. He looks pained. There is great sadness and grief in his eyes. Even though I know it is me, I don't recognise myself.

From deep within, a new thought keeps resurfacing. By now I am so tired that there is nothing I would rather want than peace and quiet. The ultimate peace and quiet. I want to disappear.

MELTDOWN

In the summer of that year the Netherlands is plunged into mourning for days on end because of the major flight MH17 air disaster in the Ukraine.

The news is dominated by it, but I can't take it all in. I am not doing well. I am not doing well at all. During the summer, I have been getting increasingly depressed. I am isolating myself and balance on the limits of my abilities. It won't take a lot for the ground to give way.

I am sitting on the sofa with my wife and my kids and we are watching television together. On the 23rd of July, at ten to four in the afternoon, the first 40 coffins, carrying the victims of the MH17 plane shot down over the Ukraine are offloaded at an air base. One by one the coffins are carried from the planes by soldiers, with huge respect and reverence. I watch what is happening live on the television, but I feel the images of the ceremony in Kandahar. It is as if I am at the ceremony again for the six fallen Canadian brothers we couldn't save. It hits me with such brute force that I am extremely upset. My wife quickly changes the channel.

I am not going to be able to stay upright. My depression is getting more severe. I thought I had hit rock bottom last year, but when I look down now, all I see is more black. I can't actually see the bottom, but I know I am on my way without being able to stop myself. Slowly but surely the last pieces of solid ground are crumbling under my feet.

I have started to fall.

❧

Two weeks later I am at our holiday address with my family and I am the worst company ever. Every single day I just sit on a chair as I am staring into the distance without uttering a single word. All my energy is gone. I don't feel like doing anything and that makes me hate myself even more. I feel useless. Again, I haven't been able to keep standing, haven't asked for help on time and I am a burden to everyone. I am deserting my family once again and I can't take it anymore.

Why the hell did I even think that I was going to be able to keep going for four months without help of Jeff whatsoever? I am going mad. No, I already am mad.

After the holiday I still can't find any peace. Even though I am exercising and walking a lot, I can't empty my head. It makes me feel despondent and worse than ever and I often feel like nothing matters anymore. I am trying so hard, but I can't do it. I am being overtaken by the past. I am done and I want it all to be over. It can all be over as far as I am concerned.

At times I take stock of my life, and list all the things I have experienced. Both the beautiful and the awful ones. Are there any reasons for me to keep fighting? I think about that more and more during my walks. Is it all worth it?

I have been going over old ground for a year now. When I started talking, I felt like I was going to win this fight. I am not so sure about that now. Every now and again I think it would be easier if I would just leave it all.

~

I reach a new low in August. I have been feeling down all day. I ring Marty, an ex-colleague and doctor, hoping that he is able to help me get some calming tablets. I need them.

Unfortunately, I can't reach him by phone and it stresses me out so much that I walk out of the door without saying a word.

It is dark. I walk with big steps. Cars are rushing by me and with every car that passes I hope the driver doesn't pay attention for just one moment and will hit me. That would be a good solution. The thought scares me, but I can feel that I actually mean it. I don't feel like going on like this any longer and repeatedly ask myself the question if I want to die. Reluctantly I have to admit that this is the case. Have I sunk so goddamn deep that I actually want to call it a day?

As I am walking I ring Marty once more, leaving him a voicemail message. I keep going along the busy road and stop to have a look at the level crossing.

I see a train hurtling past at top speed. Why don't I have an emergency number for immediate help? Through a Veterans' site I get through to an aid worker on the lowest tier, and I tell him I am wandering around. I agree with him that I will walk home and I have to promise him that I won't hurt myself. When I get home, I drink far too much alcohol, for the first time in a long time. I drink to forget.

Marty phones me at eight o'clock in the morning. I tell him openly that I don't like myself anymore.

"Well, then we have a fundamental difference of opinion, because I do like you," he jokes.

I smile briefly.

Quickly he turns serious again and tells me these are serious signals which need to be acted upon. He is going to get in touch with the Military Mental Health Department straight away and will arrange an emergency appointment for me.

Within minutes, he rings me back to say that I can go and see Jeff, who is back from deployment, in three days' time.

The next couple of days are truly horrendous and I can't do anything but sit in the garden and walk away regularly. I cry as I am walking through my neighbourhood and I can't get rid of the ever growing feeling that I want to die.

A few days later I am in the waiting room at the Military Mental Health Department, trembling and crying as I am waiting for Jeff.

This fight is breaking me, very slowly and painfully. My conversation with him is exhausting and this time I put all my cards on the table in one and a half hours. I tell him about all that bothers me, that I am still not doing well and that I don't like myself anymore. I really need help now.

He says it is a good idea for me to speak to a psychiatrist straight after this talk, as he will be able to help me find much needed peace and quiet. He says that my desire for peace means that my body and soul long for the ultimate peace, and that a passive death wish can indeed develop like that.

I talk to the psychiatrist for another hour and leave with a prescription for a shitload of medication. It is time for several sleeping pills and antidepressants and something to calm me down.

FALLING

I pour myself a fresh cup of coffee, but nearly as much coffee ends up next to the mug as in it. My hands shake heavily, as they have been doing for weeks. I curse out loud and put the pot back on the coffee maker with a bang. I sigh. I feel I have really lost control over myself and now also over the easiest of actions like pouring a cup of coffee.

When I am not sitting quietly in a chair, staring absentmindedly into the distance, I am roaming around outside. Every time I hope I can clear my head by walking. It worked quite well initially, but it doesn't anymore. How much longer can I keep fighting?

My laptop hums softly on the garden table. The screen displays an empty document. Next to the computer is my little diary. The hard cover is pale green and looks a bit grubby. I can't remember the last time I slept for more than three hours in a row. Covered in sweat I wake up numerous times during the night. I then get out of bed, so that my wife can sleep peacefully.

During the day I sit and stare for hours, eyes glazed over. I am reliving memories, deep in thought and experience flashbacks. They are all so lifelike and scare me to death. I am hyper alert and extremely tense, as restless and agitated feelings race through my body all day long.

The victims that we operated in the desert of southern Afghanistan, come by one by one. It has been seven years, but it still feels like I am there every day. For years I have avoided and fled the memories, denying what happened and pushing away every single thought about it.

I keep on staring at the empty document on my laptop. Then I shake my head and close the computer. On the opened page of my green notebook I read my scribbled down words: 22nd August: shit day! The worst one yet.

I close the book and throw it in the garden.

"How it was over there? Hot. Boiling hot and very busy." My standard reply to the question of how it was in Afghanistan. I am quiet for a bit, but my silence is soon broken by a sob - mine.

"I want it to stop. I don't want this anymore!" When I look up, I see the worried faces of my wife and my mum. Tears well up in my eyes and the first one makes its way down my cheek. My lips taste salty when I wet them with my tongue. I try and roll another cigarette with my shaky hands. The previous one is still smouldering in the ashtray. I am falling.

REUNION

It is a dreary Sunday afternoon. I have arranged to meet up with Linda. I haven't spoken to her in years, but today I am going to see her to tell her I am going mad, or that I have already gone mad.

A few days ago I rang her, because she is really the only one who can almost guess what I am thinking.

To her I will be able to say: "Do you remember that time when…", and then she will nod her head. With her I experienced immensely difficult things and I really want to speak to her. She will understand me.

As soon as she opens the door I see her heartwarming smile. She takes a step towards me and hugs me tight.

"Linda, darling, seven years, but you haven't aged a day!" I say with a smile, and I feel a first tear roll down my cheek.

"Suck-up!" she says smiling, as she walks ahead of me into the house. Once inside I start to tell her about what has been happening to me lately. She listens while she feeds me one after the other cup of tea and chocolate too.

We sit together on the wooden garden bench in her front garden. It is chilly and it starts to drizzle. I am trembling, but not because of the cold. Linda has put a blanket over our legs and a big mug of tea is cooling on the arm of the bench. She watches me with a concerned look in her eyes as big tears continue to roll down my cheeks. With shaking hands I smoke one cigarette after another. While crying I tell her that our bond is the only positive thing that I have left from my time in Afghanistan. "I'm sorry, Linda. I've had it. My bucket is full and is over spilling. I have had enough of it. I hate myself and I have to stop myself from killing the guy I see staring back at me in the mirror every morning. I wish I was dead."

LOOKING BACK

I have been scared to fall asleep for quite some time now. I am frightened of the flashbacks that come every night and I haven't slept properly for weeks. Falling asleep isn't too hard, but every single night I wake up in a cold sweat after only an hour. I often see the little boy with the knife in his head, or the boy whose leg we took off and when I think about them I am angry and sad all over again.

When I write about all the events in Afghanistan as part of my therapy I often want to stop. It is as if I can't go on. During those moments it is too painful to go back to it all. I am not able to put into words what I feel, and if I am honest I don't really want to anyway. What good does it do to tell the outside world about these horrors?

I switch on my nightlight. Recently I have been keeping a little notebook on my nightstand, in which I write the thoughts that are in my head when I wake up. The pages are completely covered in illegible and incoherent key words. I hear my wife's deep, regular breathing. I add another couple of thoughts to paper.

It is the middle of the night, the moon is high in the sky and lights up the neighbourhood. I get dressed and quietly close the front door behind me. I pull up my collar against the cold and damp and I start to walk my usual route through the housing estate.

Trembling I sit down in the kitchen over an hour later. I am freezing. There is a cup of tea on the dining table, it fogs up my reading glasses. My laptop is next to it. I hold my green diary and leave through it absentmindedly. Before my deployment I had planned to jot down all sorts of fun, hilarious and impressive anecdotes for those who stayed behind. Sadly that didn't happen. It became a factual list of sickening cases. A bit further on in the diary there are some pages with more than just an overview of our surgery patients. This is where I bluntly give my opinion about the country and all that happens there.

My handwriting looks shaky. When I see my notes I feel just like I did when I wrote them down. I find the page I am looking for. There is not a lot of writing on it. What it does say though is that everyone tells me that I was losing so much weight. That is happening again. I am losing weight quickly, probably because of an unhealthy dose of stress combined with lots of exercise.

The only thing that completely empties my head is judo and exercising. Controlled fighting on the mat till the bitter end, with respect for each other, is a good outlet. Other than during judo I now also feel that I fight till the bitter end with myself every single day.

All conversations with my psychologist Jeff, all the writing I do and all the reliving and flashbacks make that I am in the middle of the war once again. It is as if it all happened yesterday.

The pain is as intense now as it was back then. I really hope I am able to get rid of the sharp edges before I fight myself to death.

I turn a couple of pages of my diary. Shivers run down my spine and I gasp for air. The day I have to try and describe soon is one I will struggle with a lot. I worry that I won't be able to put words to paper without having a mental breakdown.

How will I ever release my biggest fears from my head and write about that day? Where do I start? The feeling that comes up when I think about that day is like one big, dark, threatening cloud. This is the day I felt frightened to death for the first time ever. That fear stayed with me for the rest of my deployment. I read out loud: "Attacked."

ONE LAST GOODBYE

I was able to write down the first couple of weeks of my deployment relatively easily, as it was about the easy part of the deployment, apart from a couple of black days. The further I get, the harder it gets. Writing about it makes me relive every day. The more I get pulled back to Afghanistan, the more I feel I have failed. The more I put pen to paper to write down each detail, and every feeling I had over there, the more I detest myself. I have been silent for seven years and have cheated myself and my family by doing so. I am absolutely furious and despise myself.

The dark clouds in my head are growing. I am slowly becoming afraid of myself and I am now facing a dilemma. Why would I continue with this battle? I am scared of this dark side and frightened to death that I will lose control of myself.

This time I have to wade through this pool of misery and no longer walk around it. The pool is deep and I hope I will be able to hold my head above water long enough to keep breathing. Once I have reached the deepest part I will be able to put my feet on the bottom again and slowly crawl out of it. This is the road I want to, have to and will take.

I really hope the dark side isn't going to get the upper hand, telling me that it is okay to let myself sink to the bottom because I will be done then. I wrestle with it every day.

My medication is increased rapidly. It is hell every time that is done. A common symptom is, that during the time it takes for the increased medication to have its effect, the complaints worsen. This period usually lasts six to eight weeks. Every single time this period is all about one thing and one thing only; surviving.

After a while the medication kicks in and does calm me down at night. The tense feeling is ever-present during the day though. That is also due to my writing. I dread having to write about the next days that are in the diary. Lots has happened during those days in Afghanistan that I am still struggling with. We operated patients whose faces I can still draw out in detail to this very day.

I now have to describe those surgeries, which made me feel so bad, and explain exactly how they make me feel. Should I not just let those memories rest? I don't seem to hand in my writing tasks as often anymore and I know I have to discuss that with Jeff. He can help me to deal with it.

"They won't understand anyway. They weren't there." It is my standard response. "The only one who understands me is Linda, who I worked shoulder to shoulder with and who was there with me on the floor during those missile attacks."

Jeff still advises me to tell more people about what I did in the desert. He knows I feel really bad about the deployment and about myself. According to him I automatically assume that others will feel the same.

"If you never talk to them about it, you'll never find out. You might well be pleasantly surprised. There are lots of people who really respect what you guys did over there. Just look at how many people stand at the side of the road on Veterans Day."

I promise him that I will let some people know what happened, and thus create a small circle of people around me who know.

After we have already said goodbye and I have put on my coat, I tell him that I am increasingly struggling with writing about the days and that I delay it more often. I don't tell him that I do that because I am afraid I am going to drown and lose control over myself. He reads my behaviour as a way of avoiding things and tasks me with writing at least two pieces every week. He will keep track to make sure I do enough.

I am shocked by his reaction, but smile at him and let him know that I won't disappoint him. Instead of stepping on the brake and signalling that he has misunderstood me and that I need help, because I am afraid of what is about to come, I dutifully concede. When I walk out of the door, I want to kick myself. My heart is in my throat and I am angry with myself as I get in my car.

The following Saturday I do start to write about the day I dread most. The sleeping monster called recollection is awakening. I write without any breaks and fully relive the fear, the loss and the desperation.

I haven't only woken the sleeping monster, but I have given it a kick up its bum! I cry for the rest of the day and I am really tense. Normally, I feel some sort of relief after I have written things down. This time the exact opposite happens. I am shaking like a leaf and feel really emotional. The people close to me notice it too. I am not myself and tell my family that I am afraid I have now really hit rock bottom.

At night I am trapped in a film that is repeated and which shows new details all the time. My head feels about to burst. I finally lose control. I am caught in a torrent of emotions, a whirlpool that drags me down and drowns me.

The next morning something happens that I have been afraid of. My heart is racing and it feels like there is a band around my chest that is being pulled tighter and tighter. I tell my wife that it is probably because of stress, but I do ring my GP when I start sweating and gagging a little later.

"I am a veteran with PTSD and I am not doing that well at the moment. It's probably stress, but I have all the symptoms of a heart attack."

Within a few minutes an emergency doctor arrives. He examines me and rules out a heart attack. I have resigned myself to what is happening and I sit on the sofa, impassively and unresponsively. The doctor stays with me for an hour and tries to get through to me, which he can't. He advises me to get in touch with Defence. I try to ring Jeff, but I can't get through.

Then it becomes painfully clear that I have no clue whatsoever how to get help in the weekend in case my therapist doesn't answer his phone. I have no idea if there is some sort of Military Mental Health 24-hours hotline or so. I also find out this GP doesn't really know how to deal with a veteran.

"The only thing I can do for you is refer you to the mainstream crisis centre."

I categorically refuse that. "I already have help, but I just don't know how to get through to them! I'm sorry, but you're useless!" I spit out the words at the GP who looks a little stunned. I ring the Veterans Institute and I speak to an operator who immediately makes me feel extremely aggressive. She informs me without any form of cooperation that as an existing patient I have to get in touch with my own psychologist. I say that I have of course tried that already, but that there is no answer. The operator can't or doesn't want to do anything for me. Furiously I disconnect the call.

Luckily Jeff has heard the voicemail message I left him and returns my call very quickly. I tell him I am broken, that I have taken stock and that I am completely and utterly done. He immediately gets to work and arranges that I am called back by a military service psychiatrist who can supply me with a prescription to really calm me down. He tells me that a psychiatric nurse will get in touch with me right away.

Shortly after, a soothing voice reassures me that she is there for me. She tells me that her name is Susan and that the department she works for can be contacted 24 hours a day. By anyone, including me and that I should never feel ashamed if I feel that I should call them. They would rather talk too much than miss one important call.

I am grateful and completely forget to complain about the Veterans Institute's operator, who obviously has never heard of this helpline. I apologise that I am being a pain on this Sunday, but she immediately interrupts me to tell me that they are really here 24 hours per day, every single day. I thank her from the bottom of my heart and save the number to my phone.

I go and get my medication, antipsychotics, with my mum. I immediately take some tablets. When I am at home it takes less than an hour for something to change in my head. It makes me calmer and flatter. It is wonderful, but it does not erase my death wish.

"It happened, dude. I hit rock bottom with a bang."

Sebastian listens as I tell him what happened to me over the last couple of days and how I am decompensating psychologically. I tell him I have gone mad and that I have started taking antipsychotics.

"I despise myself and I want to die. The only thing I want is to go and dangle from a bridge or give the first train driver I come across a very bad day. And that's exactly what I am gonna do, my friend. I just wanted to say goodbye," I say to him.

Up to that moment Sebastian has been listening, but this is when he interrupts me. "I hear what you're saying and that you're about to leave it all behind. Good for you to ring me, dude. If that happens again, give me another call. I'll drive over to stop you straight away... or to give you the last little push."

I can't help but laugh. He turns serious quickly again though and I can hear in his voice that he is really concerned. "Erik, you have regrets about seven years ago. Damn, let's make sure that you don't have any regrets about today in seven years."

Standing with the phone in my hand and smoking another cigarette, I fall silent. Then I look inside and I see my wife and two boys sitting on the sofa. They are watching television and I can see tension on all of their faces. I suddenly realise I had almost given up on them. I promise Sebastian to go inside and to get rid of my farewell letter and to go to bed.

Every time I go through a bad period, I think about his words on that cold Sunday evening, when I was so heavily medicated and about to kill myself. I am deeply grateful.

～

For the first time in ages I sleep for nine hours straight.

I take my medication for another few days and I am calmer. The tablets make me feel flat. I see all the misery pass by in my head, but I don't feel anything with it.

Unfortunately, it is only temporary. During the days that follow the treatment with the psychologist and psychiatrist is intensified. We thoroughly discuss the misunderstanding caused by me when I didn't point out that it was getting too tough for me. The longer the treatment, the closer we get to my own core.

We discuss the feeling that I broke during my deployment, that I failed because of that, and the feelings of shame and grief I still have when I think about some of my patients. I also talk in depth with Jeff about the coping mechanisms I have made my own and that I need to work on those.

The last couple of weeks of the year go by quickly.

Gradually, the treatments and the many conversations about the deployment and myself make that some of the jigsaw pieces fit together. The images I see have become more bearable because of the ongoing EMDR therapy and the sessions.

Other than my experiences I talk a lot about how I have changed since my deployment, and about the feelings of pride and shame. My self-image has been badly damaged because of all the traumatic experiences. The deployment happened to me, but the way I dealt with it was up to me.

CROSSING BOUNDARIES

Today I have a talk with my psychologist Jeff about blurring of moral standards and generalisation.

Once in a while I still feel extremely bad about that. Although it is common knowledge that a morbid sense of humour during the hardest moments is a coping and survival mechanism, instinctively I have sometimes gone too far.

Where is the boundary between survival and blurring of moral standards? I notice that I have developed an almost morbid feeling for harsh humour and on top of that I also generalise a lot.

I was barely able to enjoy the moment when the baby was born on that night in Kandahar. I witnessed the start of a new life, but all I could see in my head were the possible atrocities he could commit. To me it was certain that this boy would belong to the next generation that would be carrying out the same barbaric acts as the generations before him.

"He'll be eight years old now, Jeff," I say to the psychologist. "Would he still be alive?"

I take a sip of coffee from the carton cup. It is ice cold and I pull a disgusted face.

Jeff bursts out laughing. I laugh too.

~

The generalising didn't stop. Over the years I have developed a distrust of people in a crowded place, for example an airport or a busy event. I tend to look over my shoulder to search for suspicious people. Someone with an explosive belt might suddenly appear.

I expect that something bad is about to happen at all times. If the aim of terror is to spread fear amongst people, then they have been successful in my case. Although I don't feel good about it, it has slowly crept in and won't leave just yet.

Even though I have learnt that everyone is equal, regardless of gender, race and orientation, it has been slightly differentiated in my head. I will have to have many more conversations about this with Jeff.

I am not proud of how I laughed and joked in the operating room in Afghanistan at the expense of patients. I have made extremely harsh statements about injuries. I have spoken at length about this with the psychologist and I have asked myself many times: did I behave within the normal limits or did I cross boundaries? Did I go too far?

According to him it is a good sign that I consciously think about my functioning. I was moved by patients, even during the hardest of days. That is proof that I wasn't completely numb back then and that I didn't carry on as an insensitive robot. I apparently needed that morbid humour to survive.

The fact it still moves me after all those years and that I am so conscious about it shows that I haven't fallen prey to blurring of moral standards, but that I have fought as hard as I could to survive.

MORAL INJURY

It is a rainy October morning when I am at the psychologist where I discuss at length that one fateful evening with the interpreter.

I need a lot of breaks and I find the conversation extremely difficult. It has taken a long time and many EMDR sessions before I was even able to talk about this day. Jeff has helped me to get to the very core.

This day forms the base of my PTSD. It was on that sweltering August night in 2007 that a number of things came together and hit me with full force. It added to the misery of all the previous days.

"Start again, please," Jeff says.

Once again, I have to describe in detail what is going on inside of me, as I fill one tissue after another. "I felt lonely and abandoned, and you know what, I still do. Almost everyone immediately walked away from the patient. I am still angry about the fact we couldn't save him and I blame myself for it. I am sad, because it was a guy I could identify with."

I regarded the interpreter as an aid worker, just like myself. He was around my age. Would he have had two boys at home who were waiting for him? They would have had to process the news that daddy wasn't going to come home ever again.

"Thank goodness I performed a bit better on that front," I try jokingly, but I am not smiling.

After long conversations with Jeff I now know that I had been shaken to the core during my deployment. That happened, for example, during the first attacks, when I was frightened to death and I was certain that I would die. These blasts - they were so close. The ground trembled under my feet and I was pretty sure that the next one would hit me.

I wasn't going to leave Afghanistan alive. I would also be carried off in a coffin and there would be an honour guard formed by colleagues during a ramp ceremony. Amazing Grace would be played on the bagpipes and I would be placed in the belly of a transport plane that would take me back home, where my wife and children would be waiting for me with tearstained faces.

I was severely hurt on the night when the interpreter lost his life. That day my self-image crumbled to a little pile of rubble. My reconstruction will take years. I couldn't save him. The only thing I could do was fetch extra supplies. After he became an angel, I closed the body. I stitched up the huge wounds and I feel really bad about that. It feels as if I had to clear up the mess after we failed, after I failed. I still feel the pain every time I think of this patient. I tell myself that I shouldn't feel like that, because loss is also a part of the job in an OR room. Most patients make it, and some don't.

Rationally I can cope with it, but the heart says different things to me. But there is such a big difference between working at a surgery department of a well-equipped western hospital and performing surgery under war conditions in a desolate desert. In a western hospital, only the surgical area remains visible of a patient who is not visible as a complete human being. Performing surgery in conditions like they were back in Afghanistan is so different. If need be, the casualty is placed on the table in his own clothes, which are often shot to pieces or cut open.

That night we immediately started to try and save the interpreter's life. He was on that table in his own clothes. A young person in the prime of his life that was damaged intentionally. A man I could identify with.

These aspects and the dramatic outcome of that particular evening make that I had to deal with the full force of the load. This came on top of weeks filled with too many impressions and not enough rest.

This is how I got my second injury. A wound that used to and still goes deeper than just a memory. It is a wound deep within the core of my being.

The psychologist tells me that the process of treatment was like peeling back the layers of the onion. Most experiences in the desert have been stored in the outer layers. We peeled those away together, layer by layer and now that the outer layers have been removed we are getting closer to the core.

"Besides PTSD it looks like you are suffering from a *moral injury*." He explains that it is the psychological damage military personnel may develop during their deployment because of traumatic experiences in combination with moral dilemmas. In short, it means that I have done things that go against my own values. It goes hand in hand with feelings of guilt, shame, regret and despair. I recognise all of them, on top of the PTSD symptoms.

A long talk follows, during which Jeff writes down some black-white statements on a big whiteboard. They are all supposed to challenge and provoke me. He has done it again. Every statement hits me. I am a bad person, he writes on the board and then he underlines it. Then he tells me that that sentence explains what I feel about myself.

I am fuming. I look at him angrily and spit out a torrent of words. What does he actually think of me? Me, who is always there for his fellow human being and who relentlessly sacrifices himself in favour of others. "I always set the bar extremely high for others, but never as high as I put it for myself!" I bite. "You have probably noted that down somewhere in my file, bloody moron! What are you trying to achieve?"

Then he breaks through my hastily put up armour with a couple of well-aimed comments and after only half an hour I admit as I am sobbing that I am an awful and bad person. I acted contrary to my own moral judgment and that has hurt me even more.

Since the start of my therapy I have been able to give the events that have led to my PTSD a place, to some extent at least and rather slowly. Even though I am happy with that, I still feel taken aback by what he just said. So, there is a lot more wrong with me, and I know I have to address that. Dealing with the memories is only chapter one. We will now turn this page and write the next page. "I fear that we are stuck with each other for quite some time, Jeff."

LESSON LEARNED

Several moments during my time in Afghanistan contributed to my PTSD. During the preparation there was a lot of room for differences in perception. After the initial prep course I was under the impression that we would be sent to a sunny place where we would perform some surgery once in a while, but my colleague thought we would end up in a true hell on earth and would come back all messed up.

Ideally, there would not have been any ambiguity about what medics expect when they are deployed to work in such primitive circumstances. We should have been better prepared for war victims. Perhaps it would have been wise for the surgical teams to work, before our deployment, in places with more cases like those you would find in war zones. These could be big, foreign trauma centres for example.

Personally, I thought it was hard to be part of a small team of people without much common ground. A team that was pieced together and put on a plane to perform surgery thousands of miles away.

I often had the feeling that I wasn't part of a bigger unit. It seemed like we were on our own a lot. Officially we were part of the TFU-3: *Task Force Uruzgan*, but we had little to no contact with this parent task force. TFU was mainly stationed at Tarin Kowt in the neighbouring province of Uruzgan and at the outposts, whereas we were working at Kandahar Airfield in the province of Kandahar.

We were lucky that as a team we were quickly embraced by our air force colleagues of the ATF, the *Air Task Force*. More than once these colleagues were there to immediately help us when we had questions.

Something that I still think about a lot is the way I came back. It only became clear at the last moment that we wouldn't be flown out to Crete for adaptation days. This is a wasted opportunity. I am not under the illusion that those two days in Crete would have changed everything, but the fact we didn't have the chance to go there seems a major shortcoming. There would have been an opportunity during a group talk or an individual session to already indicate that I was having a tough time. I was simply denied this chance, and arrived back home in full war mode. I have spoken to my psychologist about this at length. It is a big deal to me and in my eyes it is strange that there is uncertainty about returning home. Every deployed soldier should have this opportunity. Two days at the very least to get used to fact that the level of vigilance is allowed to drop again, but also to be able to point out whether to expect psychological issues judging by the deployed soldier's condition.

After my return it happened several more times that small, specialist teams didn't get flown back home via Crete for one reason or another.

An ex-colleague who has been deployed more than once told me that one of the reasons for a team not going to Crete was that they would be home one or two days later. A team arriving later would mean that Defence would have to compensate the hospital where that team would normally work.

So that means that financial reasons are actually given precedence over the wellbeing of deployed forces. I nearly exploded when I heard this story and I immediately raised it with my practitioner.

He is closely involved with and largely responsible for the deployment policy, and has informed me that Defence has now made sure that it is standard procedure for surgical teams to fly back via a neutral location, and that they will have adaptation days too. I think it is a good thing and a real lesson learned.

BREAK THE SILENCE

When I came back home and people asked me how it was over there in Afghanistan, I would jokingly say that I could write a book about it. I always knew it would never be an exciting boys' book. It is a story about the other side of war. About the suffering of the wounded, intentionally or unintentionally. About the extreme pressure, and my gradual breakdown.

There are many more medics who have experienced traumatic events and don't know how to deal with it, who are ashamed to ask for help or who are as stubborn as I am not to ask for it. I hope that through my story I am able to reach even just one person who recognises her- or himself in it. I hope that my story can contribute to preventing unnecessary misery. Maybe even help save a life. Mental healthcare exists for a reason.

It is down to the person in question though whether he or she wants to use it and is actually able to acknowledge that something is horribly wrong. It took way too long for me.

Besides publishing this book, I will continue my musical indulgences together with my friends, so we can create a musical monument alongside the story in book form. Other than that it is fun, it also works therapeutically for me.

The negative spiral that I have been in for years is carefully being broken, and I am slowly bending it towards something positive. The result of it is in your hands right now.

ACKNOWLEDGMENTS

I am grateful to so many people, that I won't be able to mention them all. For everyone I don't mention, please know that it is only so on paper and not in my heart.

First of all, I would like to thank Linda from the bottom of my heart. She stood shoulder to shoulder with me in the OR in Afghanistan. Together with her I shared the ups and downs during those long, difficult weeks in the desert and she was there for me all those years later too. She will forever have a special place in my heart.

I want to express so much warmth, love and gratitude to my best friend Sebastian and his dear wife Marilyn. Without them I wouldn't be where I am today. Sebastian is a creative man of many talents and I am proud to call him my best friend. Sebastian and Marilyn, I love you to the moon and back!

Our creative journey continues. The theatre show, based on my story, currently sells out theatres all over the Netherlands. We hope to perform our show in other countries too. This universal story touches people and moves them. It is storytelling pur sang and it is about breaking the silence! Proud to be part of our band of brothers, *7even*

Bridges: Sebastian, Danny, Fondy, Guz, Marcel and Marrin. It is an honour to be on this second part of the journey with you.

I am grateful to the Ministry of Defence. It is there where I experienced a wonderful career for fourteen years of my life. The organisation immediately stepped up to offer the help I so desperately needed. I am still receiving care and support as this book is being published. During that very first phone call they told me they would be my safety net. And they were.

I also want to sincerely thank Jeff, my psychologist and practitioner at the Military Mental Health Department. I spent so many hours with him, as I filled tissue after tissue. I have cursed him repeatedly, because he was one of the only ones to get through to me with his, sometimes extremely confrontational, conversational techniques. He often gave me the kick up my backside that I needed. I have cursed, sworn and cried, but it has been worth every single tissue.

With his clear vision and sharp tongue, Yuri has dissected my story with surgical precision and has brought it back to its core. I thank him for our conversations in Kandahar and at home. I expect him to read this and curse loudly because I failed to say something blatantly scandalous about him.

Mark has offered me a career after my time with the Ministry of Defence. I am eternally grateful to him because he, and the rest of the QRS team, have kept their faith in me.

I thank Willemijn for the pictures on the front and back cover. In a split second she was able to take the front cover photo, which is pure, honest and full of emotion and really captures the whole story. Apart from being a true professional, I am very proud that I can call you my friend. I Love you.

Also a big, warm thank you to my vocal coach and beautiful human being Lana Wolf. She is the one who helps me to literally break the silence, on stage in theatres.

I would like to express a special word of thanks to Ilona who was able to translate my story. The difficult task of not only translating my words, but also my feelings into English. Thank you for your patience and all your efforts. We are ready for the next step.

Huge thanks also to my parents, my sister, her partner and my in-laws. They were the ones that often complained about me working too much and then had to deal with me snapping at them time and again.

But by far the most warmth, love and gratitude should of course go to my family, Harriette and my children Mika and Lars. Before, during and after my deployment they have had a tough time with me. I changed from a loving husband and father into a withdrawn, stubborn and depressed man, who was impenetrable to everyone and everything around him. Although I was deteriorating, they have always had faith in me. They have always lovingly supported me, even through my darkest days. You stayed and I can't express in words how grateful I am for that. Without you I wouldn't have made it.

Dear all, I am back.

Erik Krikke

November 2017

PICTURES

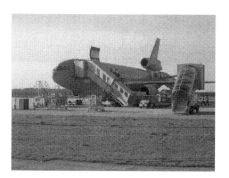

Departure from Eindhoven Airbase. The KDC-10 took us to the capital of Afghanistan, Kabul. From there we were flown to Kandahar in a Royal Air Force C-130 Hercules.

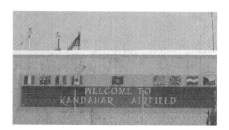

Welcome to Kandahar Airfield. The sign is attached to the TLS building, 'Taliban's Last Stand'. Legend has it that the final battles for the airport were fought here.

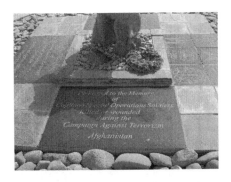

Memorial to commemorate the fallen in the fight against terrorism.

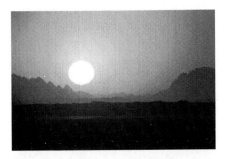

Even though Kandahar is one of the darkest places I have ever been to, the sunrise and sunset are a sight to behold.

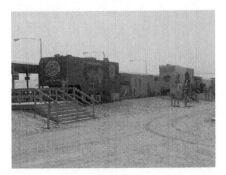

The famous food trucks at Kandahar Airfield: Burger King, Subway and Pizza Hut.

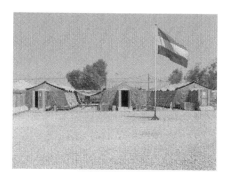

During the first days we slept in tents in the Dutch camp at Kandahar.

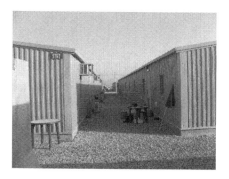

Later on we were stationed in sleeping quarters in the Canadian part of the camp.

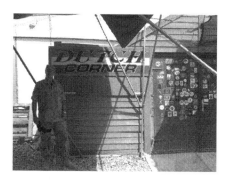

Dutch Corner; a typically Dutch place to meet for coffee, TV and games.

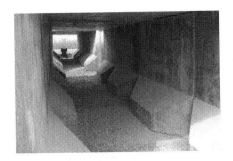

One of the many bunkers that were used to take shelter in during the numerous missile attacks.

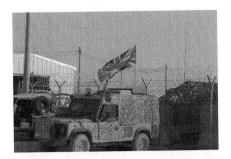

A British Landrover.

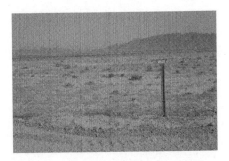

Strong advice: stay on the path. Always.

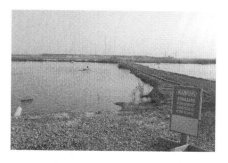

'The Shitpit' aka 'Area Fifty-Poo' aka 'The Poo Pond'.

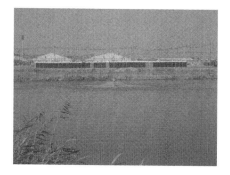

'The Shitpit' aka 'Area Fifty-Poo' aka 'The Poo Pond'.

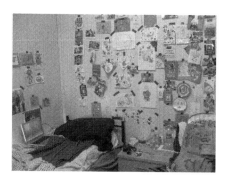

Of course I put all the post I received from home up on the wall above my bed. Every time the post arrived was a moment of pure joy.

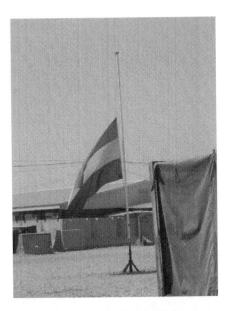

A dark day in Afghanistan: The Dutch flag is fying at half-mast.

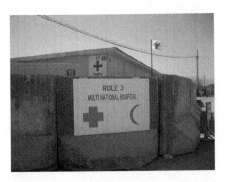

The entrance of the Role 3 MMU (Multinational Medical Unit) hospital.

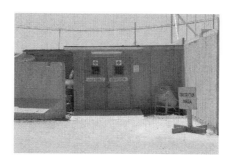

The entrance for the wounded who were brought to the hospital by helicopter.

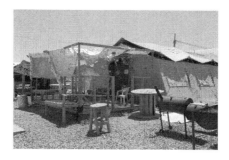

The tent behind the hospital where we could relax, looking out over the runway.

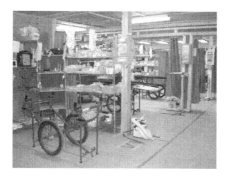

The trauma bay. Upon arrival the injured would be stabilised here first, before going into surgery.

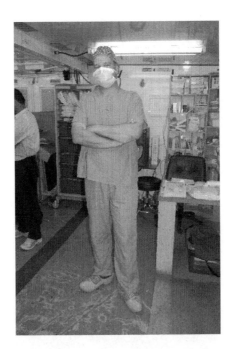

Typical...

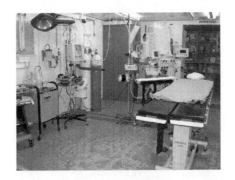

OR1 in the Role 3 MMU.

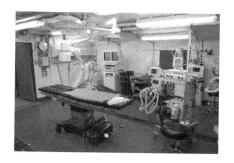

OR1 in the Role 3 MMU.

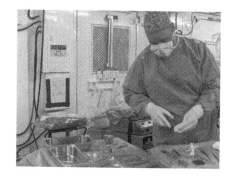

Here I am at work during one of the many surgeries.

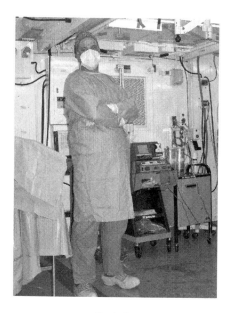

Typical...

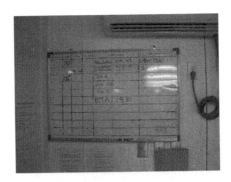

22nd August 2007. The day that would be imprinted in my soul for the rest of my life.

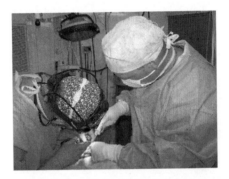

Here I am at work during during one of the many surgeries.

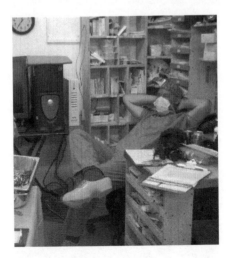

Some peace and quiet after a long day in the OR.

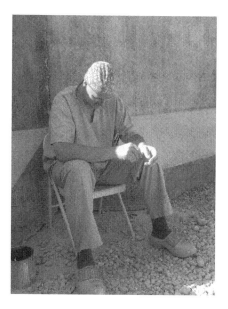

Smoking a cigarette in the shade after a long day in surgery.

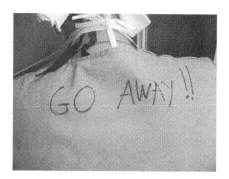

30th July. My youngest son's birthday. I couldn't be there, was grumpy, and wanted everyone to know that.

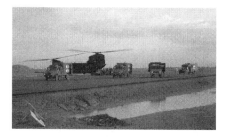

The early morning arrival of eleven wounded.

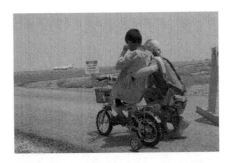

*The hospital's favourite. Brought in severely injured, but recovering
well after a long time.*

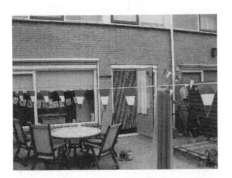

Coming home!

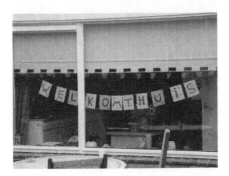

Welcome home!

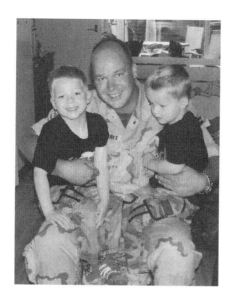

Me and my boys Mika and Lars.

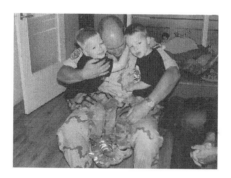

Me and my boys Mika and Lars.

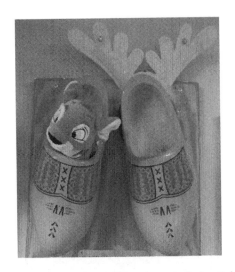

The clogs I wore in 2007 are still hanging up in the hospital. This picture was taken in 2014.

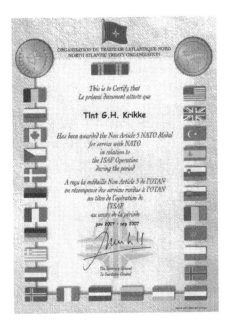

The NATO medal.

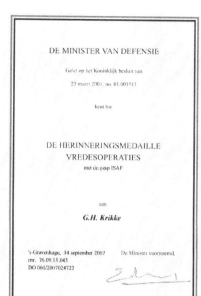

An ISAF Medal.

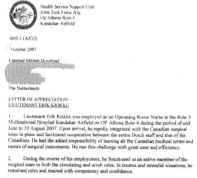

*A letter of appreciation from the commanding officers of the Role 3
Multinational Medical Unit.*

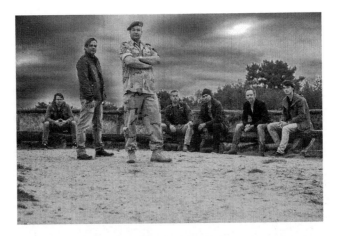

Me and my band 7even Bridges. Break the silence: We work hard to increase awareness of mental illness through our musical theatre tour and our debut album. Worldwide.

EPILOGUE

When I started writing up my notes from the diary I kept in Afghanistan, I could have never guessed that I would be making it into a story.

For me, writing about my experiences and my perception of them was part of the treatment I received for my PTSD and moral injury at the Military Mental Health Department. Only after handing in lots of writing tasks to my psychologist I slowly developed the idea to share my story. I fully realise that I have only mentioned the events in my book that I am able to tell about. There are still memories and feelings that are locked inside of me, which I cannot share at this moment and which I probably will take to my grave.

Worldwide, there are millions of veterans. I dedicate my story to all of them, young and old. Each and every one of them has devoted their life to freedom. Our own and other people's freedom.

I most definitely haven't written this book to be 'the next best literary talent', but because I have a powerful story to tell.

A story about medics not being on the frontline and yet they can get hit and hurt because of what they have been through. Members of a profession for whom suffering is seen as something 'normal' and traumatic experiences are 'the norm'.

I want to show that PTSD is a normal reaction to an abnormal situation, and that asking for help is not something to be ashamed of. In fact, being vulnerable and expressing that help is needed is sometimes the bravest thing a person can do.

Besides me, there are many aid workers and people in healthcare who experience some degree of trauma whilst they are at work.

We also shouldn't forget about their families either. My story is a universally recognisable story. It is about falling down and getting back up again.

Everybody goes through traumatic events in their lives. The question is how to deal with them. And when you fall hard and find yourself on the ground, you have always got a choice. The choice to lie down or get up. I got back up and I am grateful every day that I made that choice.

This isn't a story packed with action or excitement, but it does highlight the underexposed side of warfare. The side of the victims and of those who are there for them.

Working in a pressure cooker, under constant high pressure, as we see the most horrendous injuries, has taken its toll. The things I experienced at the hospital penetrated my soul and changed me.

I have drawn upon the notes I took during my deployment. I have also used my memories.

There are still things that are so painful I haven't been able to commit them to paper. They will be locked in my head forever. I have written about how I experienced my deployment in the only way I could: raw and personal.

APPENDIX 1: THE WAR IN AFGHANISTAN

The People's Democratic Party of Afghanistan came to power in 1978. Its regime, which was both communist and atheistic, led to the revolt of the Islamic Mujahideen, often freely translated to *holy warriors*. Because the communist regime wasn't able to control the revolt, the Soviet Union decided to support the party. When this didn't prove to be sufficient, Soviet leader Breznjev ordered the invasion of Afghanistan in 1979.

The Mujahideen strongly opposed this and they found themselves supported by, amongst others, the CIA. Once the Soviet troops retreated from Afghanistan at the end of the 1980s, the Mujahideen fell apart. The mutual enemy had been banished after all. In the period that followed the withdrawal of the Soviet troops the Mujahideen would mainly battle with one another. Different tribes and their warlords tried to seize power.

In 1994 a new group rose, the *Taliban*. Taliban is the plural of talib, which literally means *theology student*. The Taliban study at strict Koranic schools, the so-called *madrassahs*. During the Soviet invasion lots of Afghans fled to the neighbouring country of Pakistan. Besides Koran education these refugees also received free shelter and food.

These students of the *madrassahs* took charge of the Taliban during the civil war in Afghanistan which followed the withdrawal of the Soviet troops.

Soon after their rise in 1994, Kandahar was occupied by the Taliban. This city continued to be the Taliban regime's capital up to 2001. They started the battle of obtaining power over large parts of the country from the south east of Afghanistan. It wasn't until 1996 when the capital of Kabul was taken. Only the far north east of Afghanistan stayed out of the Taliban's hands. That is where the Northern Alliance ruled. Under the leadership of Mullah Mohammed Omar the Taliban subjected Afghanistan to a strict Islamic regime.

After the attacks on the 11th of September 2001, for which the terrorist group Al-Qaeda was responsible, it didn't take long for coalition forces to invade Afghanistan. This invasion wasn't trying to enforce the extradition of Osama bin Laden, but to overturn the Taliban regime. After all, the Taliban offered Al-Qaeda a safe haven. The Taliban were forced out of Kandahar in December 2001.

At the end of 2001 the Taliban were further driven out of Afghanistan. There were heavy battles between the Taliban and local warriors at the airport. At the end of 2001, just before Christmas, the airport was secured by coalition troops.

In the middle of the airport is the so-called TLS building. It stands for *Taliban's Last Stand*. Nowadays, the building serves as a passenger terminal for troops lucky enough to leave Kandahar. Legend has it that the Taliban leaders were in the building during the siege of the airport. They were able to escape at the last possible moment. They fled to the inhospitable mountains nearby.

This striking structure TLS is, has beautiful, characteristic arches and is a landmark in its own right. The building's wounds are still visible behind all the splendour. Bullet holes high up on the walls remind us of the battle that took place here over 15 years ago.

Years after my deployment I met an American plastic surgeon via social media, who was at the Role 3 hospital in Kandahar at that time. He told me that it is still busy at the hospital, but that a lot has changed since I was there. The plywood cabin from 2007 was shut down years ago and a beautiful new hospital has taken its place.

This new hospital is equipped with all comforts, is well stocked, and has more than enough staff and the admission and surgery capacity to take care of lots of victims. The walls and roof are made of reinforced concrete that is several inches thick and provide protection for the still frequent missile attacks. Even though a lot has changed, and the hospital has moved to another part of the base, my wooden clogs still hang on the wall. They are a quiet reminder of old times.

Somehow I hope the hospital has been built based on the experiences of staff like us, who worked in the old hospital. This way my bad experience would have contributed to the fact that things are well organised now. My suffering will have had a purpose.

Kandahar International Airport is located about 10 miles south east of Kandahar City. The airport was built in the 60s, with the support of the United States. It grew into the second largest airport of Afghanistan.

Today the airport has transformed into a busy military airport, called KAF, *Kandahar Airfield*. Because of the huge amount of weekly aircraft movements, Kandahar Airfield developed into the busiest airport in the world with only one runway.

All airports are designated a three-letter code. The code for Kandahar Airfield is therefore KAF. Kabul International Airport code would have been KIA, which is also the abbreviation for *killed in action*, a term no one wants to be reminded of on their outward journey. So by way of exception Kabul has a four-letter code: KAIA.

The military base of Kandahar Airfield has grown to the size of a small city. In 2012 it housed more than 26,000 personnel. The phase-out of the ISAF troops was in full swing in 2015. It won't take too long until the last ISAF troops will also leave the airport. Kandahar will then be completely handed over to the Afghan authorities.

The NATO-led ISAF mission formally ended in December 2014, after more than thirteen years. Even though the mission has finished, the violence continues. NATO has started the Resolute Support Mission with the objective to train and support Afghan security forces.

Since the ISAF mission finished the Taliban have invaded more areas of Afghanistan. Large parts of the Helmand and Kandahar provinces are now once again controlled by the Taliban. The province of Uruzgan, which was the main focus of the Dutch deployment during the ISAF mission, is the site of regular battles too and where the Taliban appear to be gaining ground.

Fights between the Taliban and the Afghan forces and police are commonplace in almost every part of the country.

The USA has recently announced plans to increase the number of American troops in Afghanistan, as the Afghan forces have suffered large losses against the Taliban, resulting in a rapidly worsening security situation.

APPENDIX 2: ROLE ASSIGNMENT

The term 'role' or 'echelon' is used to describe the four levels that organise the medical support. Treatments can be performed, evacuation can be taken care of, supplies can be provided, and other essential functions can be carried out for the maintenance and conservation of the deployability of the troops. 'Role' is mainly used for land and air forces, whereas 'echelon' is more of a maritime expression. Even though the terms are closely related, they don't actually mean the same. The concept of 'role' is explained more thoroughly below.

The possibilities in terms of treatments of each role are also an intrinsic part of the subsequent higher level. This means that a Role 3 setting has the ability to fulfil all the functions of a Role 2. Furthermore, each level in the chain of medical care has the responsibility to supply and otherwise support the lower levels. It is not a necessity for a patient to pass through every level in the chain during treatment or evacuation.

~

Role 1 medical support is usually connected or assigned to a small military unit. It can provide essential first aid, take lifesaving action and carry out triage. On top of that a Role 1 will contribute to the health and welfare of the unit by assisting in disease prevention, treatment of non-combat related conditions and guidance of operational stress. Regular surgery hours and the treatment of sick or wounded personnel with focus on the immediate return to the unit are the functions of this level of healthcare. An example of a Role 1 could be a medical centre on a military base, with normal surgery hours.

~

Role 2 support is usually given to a larger unit, often the size of a brigade or bigger. The Role 2 is able to operate in more forward positions, depending on the operational requirements. In general, this facility will be equipped to provide the evacuation of patients from Role 1 facilities. Role 2 is able to offer triage, ventilation, and resuscitation, and the nursing of patients until they are able to be evacuated or return to their unit. It also has a department for urgent dental treatments.

A Role 2 would normally not include any surgical capacity, but due to certain military operations it is often required to increase the treatment options to be able to carry out urgent surgeries and essential postoperative management. If this is the case though, the term Role 2+ is used. An example of this would be the Dutch Role 2+ at Tarin Kowt in Uruzgan.

~

Role 3 medical care is normally offered at the level of a division or bigger. It includes many extra possibilities, amongst which are specialist diagnostic resources, specialist surgical capacities and medical care, preventative medicine, food inspection, dental care, and operational stress management teams, in case they aren't provided by level 2. The intake capacity of a Role 3 facility needs be at such a level that it is able to provide diagnosis, treatment and admission of patients who need overall treatment and who will then return to active service, within the specified evacuation policy.

Role 3 medical care is normally provided by different types of field hospitals. An example of this is the Role 3 Multinational Medical Unit at Kandahar Airfield. Support of and supply to the lower levels wasn't uncommon during my deployment. There was regular contact between the Role 2+ at Tarin Kowt and the Role 3 at Kandahar. It often happened that we supplied them with extra medical resources. We would fly these out to Uruzgan.

∼

Role 4 medical care offers definitive care for patients whose essential treatment would take longer than the evacuation policy allows, or for whom the medical possibilities of a Role 3 aren't sufficient. Normally, this would include highly specialised surgical procedures, revalidation and longterm care. This level of care would usually be very time-consuming and therefore offered in their country of origin.

Examples of Role 4 care are the LRMC, *Landstuhl Regional Medical Centre*, in Germany, and the Walter Reed Hospital in the United States. After the initial life and limb saving surgical procedures at Kandahar Airfield many ISAF victims are flown out to Landstuhl to receive definitive treatment, before they are repatriated.

THANK YOU

Writing this book has been a gift to me. I started writing down all my memories and experiences as part of my treatment at the Military Mental Health Department. Eventually I chose to make it into a book and publish it, hoping it would reach even just one person. One single person who would read my book, recognise themselves in it and find the strength to ask for help and to keep going.

As soon as the book was published, I received an enormous amount of responses. Thousands of people around the world have taken the time to read my story, write a review or send me a message through social media. I personally read every comment and message. They often give me goosebumps and move me to tears. I am extremely grateful that so many people let me know that my book has touched and inspired them.

I committed my story to paper and now also share it through music, together with my band 7even Bridges. When words fail, music speaks. During the darkest times I looked for and found support in music, and now, together with my best friends, I tell my story of falling down and getting back up again.

Our album 'Break the Silence' intends to do exactly that. It is now available to download and stream.

Break the silence. I am so grateful that I have broken the silence. My story needs to be told and should be heard.

I would really appreciate it if you would write a review too.

Thank you so much!

Erik Keilie.